PROGRAMMED
MATHEMATICS
OF DRUGS
AND SOLUTIONS

PROGRAMMED MATHEMATICS OF DRUGS AND SOLUTIONS

6TH EDITION

Virginia Poole Arcangelo, PhD, FNP

Associate Professor
Department of Nursing
College of Health Professions
Thomas Jefferson University
Philadelphia, Pennsylvania

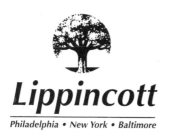

Lippincott

Philadelphia • New York • Baltimore

Editor: Margaret Zuccarini
Editorial Assistant: Helen Kogut
Production Editor: Jeffrey S. Myers
Design Coordinator: Mario Fernandez

Copyright © 1999 Lippincott Williams & Wilkins

351 West Camden Street
Baltimore, Maryland 21201-2436

227 East Washington Square
Philadelphia, PA 19106

Printed in the United States of America

Fourth Edition, 1984
Fifth Edition, 1992

Library of Congress Cataloging-in-Publication Data

Arcangelo, Virginia Poole.
   Programmed mathematics of drugs and solutions. — 6th ed. /
Virginia Poole Arcangelo.
     p. cm.
   Includes bibliographical references and index.
   ISBN 0-7817-1875-9
   1. Pharmaceutical arithmetic Programmed instruction.
I. Arcangelo, Virginia Poole. Weaver & Koehler's programmed
mathematics of drugs and solutions. II. Title.
     [DNLM: 1. Pharmaceutical Preparations—administration & dosage
Nurses' Instruction. 2. Pharmaceutical Preparations—administration
& dosage Programmed Instruction. 3. Mathematics Nurses'
Instruction. 4. Mathematics Programmed Instruction. QV 18.2 A668p
1999]
RS57.A73 1999
615'.1'01513—dc21
DNLM/DLC
for Library of Congress   99-25478
                                      CIP

To purchase additional copies of this book, call our customer service department at **(800) 638-3030** or fax orders to **(301) 824-7390**. International customers should call **(301) 714-2324**.

99 00 01 02 03
1 2 3 4 5 6 7 8 9 10

The author and the publisher would like to acknowledge the contributions of Mabel E. Weaver, RN, MS, Professor Emeritus, and Vera J. Koehler, RN, MN, Professor Emeritus, both of the Division of Nursing at California State University, Sacramento, to the original edition of this text.

PREFACE

It is essential that every individual involved in administering drugs to patients be aware of correct methods to calculate dosage. This book is designed both as a self-paced introductory program to the mathematics of drugs and solutions and as a refresher for knowledge previously learned. It provides a review of basic arithmetic and application of those concepts related to drugs and solutions. The book can be helpful to anyone responsible for administration of medications.

The reader's knowledge is tested at various points. A pretest is included to provide guidelines to areas of weakness in basic arithmetic. Numerous practice problems throughout the book provide an immediate measure of the reader's understanding of the concept presented. A comprehensive examination is included at the end of the book.

All drugs mentioned in the book have been reviewed for current use. Practice problems have been included directly after the concept discussed.

VIRGINIA POOLE ARCANGELO, PhD, FNP

TO THE READER

One important part of nursing practice is the correct administration of drugs and solutions to patients. In providing a person with the correct dosage, the nurse may need to do some mathematical calculations because the available drug may be stated in a different system of measurement or may be more or less than the amount that has been ordered. The goal of this book is to enable you to solve such problems.

To do this, mathematical concepts are presented in a practical way within the text. These concepts are then applied to the preparation of drugs and solutions. It is your responsibility to learn the mathematical skills necessary to administer medications accurately.

The names of drugs found in the problems and examples are currently used in practice. A section on proper selection and use of syringes is included.

This is a programmed textbook. It may be different from books you have used in the past in that the text is incomplete and broken down into small units called "frames." You will complete the text by filling in words or phrases or by answering the questions. The answers can be written in the frames. Check each answer as soon as you have written it by comparing it with the correct answer, which is found to the right of the frame you have just read. As you work through the program, use the included bookmark to cover the answer column. You need not be concerned if you make a mistake. The important thing is to go back and find your error and correct it.

This text will assist you in building on your mathematical skills and enable you to apply them to the clinical setting. Good luck.

TABLE OF CONTENTS

COMMON ABBREVIATIONS

āā	_____	of each
ac	_____	before meals
AD	_____	right ear
ad lib	_____	as desired
AU	_____	both ears
AS	_____	left ear
b.i.d.	_____	twice a day
c̄	_____	with
D/C	_____	discontinue
elix.	_____	elixir
ext.	_____	extract
Fl.	_____	fluid
g (or gm)	_____	gram
gr	_____	grain
gtt	_____	drop
H.	_____	hour
h.s.	_____	hour of sleep (bedtime)
IM	_____	intramuscular
IV	_____	intravenous
kg	_____	kilogram
KVO	_____	keep vein open
I (L)	_____	liter

μg (or mcg)	_____	microgram
mg	_____	milligram
ml	_____	milliliter
mEq	_____	milliequivalent
NPO	_____	nothing by mouth
OD	_____	right eye
os	_____	mouth
OS	_____	left eye
OU	_____	both eyes
oz (℥)	_____	ounce
pc	_____	after meals
per	_____	by
p.o.	_____	by mouth
prn	_____	as needed
q	_____	every
q.a.m.	_____	every morning
q.d.	_____	every day
q.h.	_____	every hour
q.i.d.	_____	four times a day
q.o.d.	_____	every other day
q.s.	_____	sufficient quantity
s	_____	without
SC	_____	subcutaneous
Sig.	_____	write on label
SL	_____	sublingual
Sol.	_____	solution
ss	_____	one-half
stat	_____	right away
t.i.d.	_____	three times a day
U	_____	unit

TABLE OF EQUIVALENTS

Liquid Measurements

1,000 cc*	= 32 fluid ounces	= 1 quart
500 cc	= 16 fluid ounces	= 1 pint
30 cc	= 1 ounce	= 2 tablespoonfuls
15 cc	= 4 fluidrams	= 1 tablespoonful
5 cc	= 1 fluidram	= 1 teaspoonful
1 cc	= 15 or 16 minims	
0.06 cc	= 1 minim	= 1 drop

*cc and ml can be used interchangeably (1 cc = 1 ml)

Weights

1 kg	= 2.2 pounds
30 gm	= 1 ounce
1 gm	= grains 15
300 mg	= grains 5
60 mg	= gr 1
1 mg	$= \text{gr } \dfrac{1}{60}$

Length

2.54 cm	= 1 inch
1 cm	= 0.39 inch

Temperature Conversions

$°F = \dfrac{9}{5}$	$= \dfrac{9}{5} °C + 32°$
$°C = \dfrac{5}{9}$	$= \dfrac{5}{9} (°F - 32°)$

GLOSSARY

Ampule	small glass container for solutions; usually used for one dose then discarded
Compatible	able to mix with another substance without causing a harmful reaction
Concentration	content of contained substance in solution
Dilute	to make less concentrated
Diluent	agent used to make substance less concentrated
Electrolyte	compound that separates into charged particles when dissolved in water
Equivalent	equal in value
Generic	name of drug that identifies it by other than its trade name
Hyperalimentation	method for providing total caloric needs intravenously for the undernourished individual
Hypertonic	greater concentration than that of a solution to which it is compared
Hypodermic	inserted under the skin
Hypotonic	lesser concentration than that of a solution to which it is compared
Isotonic	same concentration as that of a solution to which it is compared
Nomogram	representation by graph, diagram, or chart of relationship between values
Parenteral	not through the alimentary canal; i.e., subcutaneous, intramuscular, or intravenous
Precipitate	deposit separated from a solution
Proprietary	any chemical or drug used in the treatment of disease if protected against free competition by patent or copyright
Ratio	relation between two similar things

Saturated	holding all that can be absorbed
Solute	substance dissolved in solution
Solvent	liquid holding another substance in solution
Stock solution	that substance available
Unit	specifically defined amount of anything subject to measurement
U.S.P.	United States Pharmacopeia—a legally recognized compendium of standards for drugs

Knowledge Self-Assessment

This pretest is designed to help you assess your knowledge of and ability to work with fractions and decimals. As you proceed through the programmed text, you will need to apply this knowledge in the calculations to arrive at the proper dosage of medication to administer to your patient.

FRACTIONS

A. Add the following and reduce all fractions to lowest terms:

1. $\dfrac{2}{3} + \dfrac{4}{5} =$

$$\dfrac{10}{15} + \dfrac{12}{15} = \dfrac{22}{15} = 1\dfrac{7}{15}$$

2. $\dfrac{1}{3} + \dfrac{1}{2} + \dfrac{5}{6} =$

$$\dfrac{2}{6} + \dfrac{3}{6} + \dfrac{5}{6} = \dfrac{10}{6} = 1\dfrac{4}{6} = 1\dfrac{2}{3}$$

3. $5\dfrac{1}{2} + 1\dfrac{1}{3} + 4\dfrac{1}{4} =$

$$5\dfrac{6}{12} + 1\dfrac{4}{12} + 4\dfrac{3}{12} = 10\dfrac{13}{12} = 11\dfrac{1}{12}$$

4. $1\dfrac{3}{4} + 5\dfrac{1}{2} + 11\dfrac{1}{16} =$

$$1\dfrac{12}{16} + 5\dfrac{8}{16} + 11\dfrac{1}{16} = 17\dfrac{21}{16} = 18\dfrac{5}{16}$$

5. $\dfrac{3}{5} + \dfrac{4}{9} + \dfrac{7}{30} =$

$$\dfrac{54}{90} + \dfrac{40}{90} + \dfrac{21}{90} = \dfrac{115}{90} = 1\dfrac{25}{90} = 1\dfrac{5}{18}$$

B. Subtract the following and reduce all fractions to lowest terms:

1. $\dfrac{5}{8} - \dfrac{1}{3} =$

$$\dfrac{15}{24} - \dfrac{8}{24} = \dfrac{7}{24}$$

2. $2\dfrac{2}{3} - 1\dfrac{3}{4} =$

$$2\dfrac{8}{12} - 1\dfrac{9}{12} = \dfrac{32}{12} - \dfrac{21}{12} = \dfrac{11}{12}$$

3. $110\dfrac{3}{33} - 35\dfrac{2}{3} =$

$$109\dfrac{36}{33} - 35\dfrac{22}{33} = 74\dfrac{14}{33}$$

4. $5\dfrac{3}{8} - 2\dfrac{1}{6} =$

$$5\dfrac{9}{24} - 2\dfrac{4}{24} = 3\dfrac{5}{24}$$

5. $6\dfrac{4}{7} - 2\dfrac{1}{3} =$

$$6\dfrac{12}{21} - 2\dfrac{7}{21} = 4\dfrac{5}{21}$$

C. Multiply the following and reduce all fractions to lowest terms:

1. $8 \times \dfrac{3}{4} =$

$$\dfrac{8}{1} \times \dfrac{3}{4} = \dfrac{24}{4} = 6$$

2. $\dfrac{11}{12} \times \dfrac{4}{5} \times 6\dfrac{1}{4} =$

$$\dfrac{11}{12} \times \dfrac{4}{5} \times \dfrac{25}{4} = \dfrac{1100}{240} = 4\dfrac{7}{12}$$

3. $6\dfrac{6}{11} \times 7\dfrac{1}{3} =$

$$\dfrac{72}{11} \times \dfrac{22}{3} = \dfrac{1584}{33} = 48$$

4. $36 \times \dfrac{5}{6} \times \dfrac{3}{8} =$

$$\dfrac{36}{1} \times \dfrac{5}{6} \times \dfrac{3}{8} = \dfrac{540}{48} = 11\dfrac{1}{4}$$

5. $6\dfrac{1}{4} \times 4 \times 3\dfrac{2}{5} =$

$$\dfrac{25}{4} \times \dfrac{4}{1} \times \dfrac{17}{5} = \dfrac{1700}{20} = 85$$

D. Divide the following and reduce all fractions to lowest terms:

1. $16 \div \dfrac{4}{5} =$

$$\frac{16}{1} \times \frac{5}{4} = \frac{80}{4} = 20$$

2. $8\dfrac{1}{8} \div \dfrac{3}{4} =$

$$\frac{65}{8} \times \frac{4}{3} = \frac{260}{24} = 10\frac{20}{24} = 10\frac{5}{6}$$

3. $8\dfrac{1}{2} \div \dfrac{9}{16} \div 8 =$

$$\frac{7}{2} \times \frac{16}{9} \times \frac{1}{8} = \frac{272}{144} = 1\frac{128}{144} = 1\frac{8}{9}$$

4. $3\dfrac{1}{7} \div 1\dfrac{7}{15} \div 2\dfrac{2}{7} =$

$$\frac{22}{7} \times \frac{15}{22} \times \frac{7}{16} = \frac{2310}{2464} = \frac{15}{16}$$

5. $50\dfrac{4}{5} \div 1\dfrac{2}{3} =$

$$\frac{254}{5} \times \frac{3}{5} = \frac{762}{25} = 30\frac{12}{25}$$

DECIMALS

A. Add the following:

    1. $2.8 + 3.4 + 6.0 =$ 12.2

    2. $21.35 + 7.06 + 0.03 =$ 28.44

    3. $0.002 + 31.6 + 8.6 + 2.23 =$ 42.432

    4. $1.653 + 21 + 6.3 + 8.22 =$ 37.173

    5. $200.62 + 9.4 + 0.003 + 20.1 =$ 230.123

B. Subtract the following:

    1. $10.392 - 8.34 =$ 2.052

2. $20.432 - 16.66 =$ 3.772

3. $10.2 - 4.819 =$ 5.381

4. $11.6 - 5.078 =$ 6.522

5. $25.635 - 20.1 =$ 5.535

C. Multiply the following:

   1. $8.2 \times 24.3 =$ 199.26

   2. $2.65 \times 0.03 =$ 0.0795

3. $4.753 \times 2.564 =$ | 12.186692

4. $1.75 \times 0.002 =$ | 0.00350

5. $10.35 \times 0.41 =$ | 4.2435

D. Divide the following:

   1. $20.3 \div 15 =$ | 1.3533

   2. $50 \div 2.5 =$ | 20

   3. $65 \div 2.5 =$ | 26

----

4. $80 \div 0.55 =$ 145.4545

----

5. $2.1 \div 0.07 =$ 30

PROPORTIONS

Solve for x:

1. $\dfrac{4}{5} = \dfrac{x}{30}$ 24

----

2. $\dfrac{13}{20} = \dfrac{x}{5}$ 3.25

----

3. $\dfrac{5}{6} = \dfrac{8}{x}$ 9.6

----

4. $\dfrac{1}{200} = \dfrac{x}{50}$

0.25

Review of Arithmetic

Calculations of drugs and solutions require a basic understanding of whole numbers, fractions, and decimals. It is helpful to review this material. This section covers the basic rules for working with fractions, decimals, and percentages. It can be used as a review for those areas in which you were weak in the pretest.

1. A fraction is a part of a whole number. It consists of a numerator, which is the top number, and a denominator, which is the bottom number.

   In the fraction $\frac{3}{4}$, 3 is

   the _____,

   and 4 is the _____.

   numerator

   denominator

2. Fractions should always be reduced to the lowest term. To do this, the numerator and the denominator are each divided by the largest number by which they are both divisible.

   In the fraction $\frac{8}{24}$, both the numerator and denominator are divisible by eight, so $\frac{8}{24}$

   = _____.

   $\frac{1}{3}$

3. To change a mixed number (a whole number and a fraction) to a fraction, the whole number is multiplied by the denominator of the fraction. This number is added to the numerator of the fraction and the sum is placed over the denominator.

$$2\frac{1}{6} = (2 \times \underline{\hspace{1cm}}) + 1.$$

6

$$\text{So } 2\frac{1}{6} = \frac{\underline{\hspace{1cm}}}{6}.$$

13

4. To change an improper fraction (a fraction whose numerator is greater than its denominator and, therefore, whose value is greater than 1) to a mixed number, the numerator is divided by the denominator. Anything that is not further divisible is expressed as a fraction.

$$\frac{13}{6} = 6\overline{)13} = \underline{\hspace{1cm}}$$

$2\frac{1}{6}$

5. To add fractions with the same denominator, add the numerators and place that sum over the denominator. The answer is reduced to the lowest term if necessary.

$$\frac{4}{7} + \frac{2}{7} = \underline{\hspace{1cm}}$$

$\frac{6}{7}$

6. To add fractions with different denominators, first find the lowest number evenly divisible by both. This is called the "lowest common denominator." Convert each fraction to the same terms by dividing the denominator into the lowest common denominator and multiplying that answer and the numerator. The answer to this is the new numerator. The numerators are then added together and placed over the lowest common denominator.

In the problem $\dfrac{1}{6} + \dfrac{3}{4}$, the lowest common denominator of $\dfrac{1}{6}$ and $\dfrac{3}{4}$

is _____ .

$$\text{Therefore, } \frac{1}{6} = \frac{}{12} \text{ and}$$

$$\frac{3}{4} = \frac{}{12} .$$

So $\dfrac{1}{6} + \dfrac{3}{4} =$ _____ .

(The fraction should be reduced to the lowest term.)

12

2

9

$\dfrac{11}{12}$

7. To subtract fractions with the same denominator, subtract the numerators and place the answer over the denominator. The answer should be reduced to the lowest term.

$$\frac{3}{4} - \frac{1}{4} = \underline{\hspace{2cm}}$$

$$\frac{2}{4} = \frac{1}{2}$$

8. To subtract fractions with different denominators, the lowest common denominator must first be found and the fractions must be converted as in frame 6. The numerators are then subtracted and placed over the lowest common denominator and reduced to the lowest term.

In the problem $\frac{5}{7} - \frac{1}{3}$, the lowest

common denominator of $\frac{5}{7}$ and $\frac{1}{3}$

is _____.

$$\frac{5}{7} = \frac{}{21}.$$

$$\frac{1}{3} = \frac{}{21}.$$

So $\frac{5}{7} - \frac{1}{3} = \underline{\hspace{2cm}}.$

21

15

7

$\frac{8}{21}$

9. To multiply fractions, multiply the numerators together. The answer is the new numerator. Then multiply the denominators; that number is the new denominator.

In the problem $\dfrac{7}{8} \times \dfrac{1}{2}$,

$7 \times 1 =$ _____.

$8 \times 2 =$ _____.

So $\dfrac{7}{8} \times \dfrac{1}{2} =$ _____.

7

16

$\dfrac{7}{16}$

10. To divide fractions, the division problem must be changed to a multiplication problem. Do this by inverting the divisor (the number to the right of the division sign) and then following the rule for multiplication. The answer should be reduced to the lowest term.

In the problem $\dfrac{1}{8} \div 3$, the 3 is

changed to _____, and the two fractions are multiplied.

$\dfrac{1}{8} \times \dfrac{1}{3} =$ _____

$\dfrac{1}{3}$

$\dfrac{1}{24}$

The following are practice problems with fractions.

11. $\dfrac{5}{6} + \dfrac{6}{6} =$

$\dfrac{11}{6} = 1\dfrac{5}{6}$

12. $\dfrac{3}{14} + \dfrac{13}{14} =$

$\dfrac{16}{14} = 1\dfrac{2}{14} = 1\dfrac{1}{7}$

13. $3\dfrac{1}{4} + \dfrac{5}{6} =$

$\dfrac{39}{12} + \dfrac{10}{12} = \dfrac{49}{12} = 4\dfrac{1}{12}$

14. $2\dfrac{5}{16} + 4\dfrac{1}{5} =$

$\dfrac{185}{80} + \dfrac{336}{80} = \dfrac{521}{80} = 6\dfrac{41}{80}$

15. $2\dfrac{2}{5} - \dfrac{3}{4} =$

$\dfrac{48}{20} - \dfrac{15}{20} = \dfrac{33}{20} = 1\dfrac{13}{20}$

16. $\dfrac{14}{15} - \dfrac{2}{3} =$ | $\dfrac{14}{15} - \dfrac{10}{15} = \dfrac{4}{15}$

17. $\dfrac{1}{12} \times \dfrac{3}{5} =$ | $\dfrac{3}{60} = \dfrac{1}{20}$

18. $\dfrac{8}{9} \times \dfrac{3}{4} =$ | $\dfrac{24}{36} = \dfrac{2}{3}$

19. $\dfrac{9}{10} \div 4 =$ | $\dfrac{9}{10} \times \dfrac{1}{4} = \dfrac{9}{40}$

20. $\dfrac{7}{8} \div \dfrac{2}{3} =$ | $\dfrac{7}{8} \times \dfrac{3}{2} = \dfrac{21}{16} = 1\dfrac{5}{16}$

21. A decimal represents a fraction whose denominator is a multiple of 10.

0.10 is the same as the fraction $\dfrac{1}{10}$.

0.01 is the same as the fraction

_____.

$\dfrac{1}{100}$

---

22. When multiplying decimals, the two numbers are treated as whole numbers. The answer must have as many numbers to the right of the decimal point as the *total* number of decimal points in the numbers being multiplied.

3.4×1.31 will have _____ numbers to the right of the decimal point.

3

$3.4 \times 1.31 =$ _____

4.454

---

23. To divide two decimals, the decimal point of the divisor is moved to the right until the number is a whole number. The decimal point of the dividend (the number to the left of the division sign) must be moved an equal number of places.

$3 \div .02 = .02 \overline{)3.00}$

$2\overline{)300} =$ _____

150

The following are practice problems with decimals.

24. $3.25 \times 7.03 =$

22.8475

25. $9.12 \times 1.25 =$

11.4000

26. $12 \div 3.2 =$

$32 \overline{)120} = 3.75$

27. $4.25 \div 3.1 =$

$31 \overline{)42.5} = 1.371$

28. The term percent (%) means parts per hundred. To change a percent to a decimal, the % symbol is dropped and the number is divided by 100.

20% is the same as the decimal

_____.

.20

29. When calculating with percentages, the % sign is dropped, the number is changed to a decimal, and rules pertaining to decimals are followed.

The following are practice problems using percentage.

30. $13 \times 20\% =$

$13 \times .20 = 2.60$

---

31. $6.2 \times 31\% =$

$6.2 \times .31 = 1.922$

---

32. $24 \div 8\% =$

$$8\overline{)2400} = 300$$

---

33. A ratio expresses the comparison of one number with another.

A ratio expressing the relationship of three to four is written with a colon between the two numbers (3:4) or as a fraction ($\frac{3}{4}$).

The ratio expressing the relationship

of 7 to 8 can be written _____ or

_____.

7:8

$\frac{7}{8}$

---

34. A proportion is a statement of two ratios that are equal. An example is

$\frac{1}{5} = \frac{20}{100}$. It is read, _____ is equal to 20 to 100.

1 to 5

---

35. One number in a proportion may be missing. The missing number is replaced by an x.

For example, $\dfrac{2}{3} = \dfrac{x}{12}$. It is necessary to find the value of x.

To find the value of x, cross multiply.

$$\dfrac{2}{3} = \dfrac{x}{12}$$

$2 \times 12 = 3x$

_____ $= 3x$ 24

$x = 24 \div 3$

$x =$ _____   8

---

36. Solve for x in the following problem.

$$\dfrac{3}{7} = \dfrac{12}{x}$$

$3x = 7 \times 12$

$3x =$ _____   84

$x =$ _____   28

The following are practice problems for proportions.

37. $\dfrac{1}{6} = \dfrac{x}{24}$

$x = 4$

38. $\dfrac{4}{9} = \dfrac{8}{x}$

$x = 18$

39. $\dfrac{3}{5} = \dfrac{x}{25}$

$x = 15$

Using the Metric System

2

The first step in learning about the mathematics of drugs and solutions is to become familiar with the various systems and units used in measuring drugs and solutions. The first of these systems is the *metric* system of weights and measures. The metric system was developed in France in the latter part of the eighteenth century and is used in most European countries. Today, the metric system is utilized in hospitals throughout the United States. In the metric system, fractional quantities (i.e., less than one) are expressed as decimals. For example, one-half is written as 0.5. In this system, the unit of length is the meter (hence "metric").

The units used in measuring medication are (1) weight—the kilogram, the gram, and the milligram; and (2) volume—the liter and the milliliter or the cubic centimeter. (Although the milliliter and the cubic centimeter are not exactly equal, the difference is so slight that the terms are used interchangeably).

This chapter will examine the relationships between these units for weight and volume and will show how quantities are expressed within the framework of the metric system.

1. When administering medications to the patient, one of three systems of measurements will be used. The first of these that we will discuss is the international decimal system called the <u>metric system</u>.

   The _____ _____ is the international decimal system of weights and measures.

   metric system

2. In the metric system, fractions are expressed as decimals. In the decimal system, the fraction one-half is written as 0.5.

   Four-tenths is written as _____.

   0.4

3. The unit of weight in the metric system is expressed in terms of the gram (g).

   The _____ is said to be the unit of weight in the metric system.

   gram

4. In the metric system, five grams is written 5.0 grams or 5.0 g.

   Ten grams is written as 10.0 g or

   _____ _____.

   10.0 grams

---

5. The prefix "kilo" indicates 1,000.0.

A kilogram (kg) is _____ grams.

| 1,000.0

---

6. To change kilograms to grams, <u>multiply</u> the number of kilograms by <u>1,000</u> or move the decimal three places to the *right*.

Thus:
5.0 kilograms (kg) × 1,000 = 5,000.0 grams (g) or
5.0 kilograms (kg) = 5.000 = 5,000.0 grams (g)

10.0 kg = _____ g

| 10,000.0

---

7. 400.0 kg = 400,000.0 g

25.0 kg = _____ g

| 25,000.0

---

8. 2.0 kg = _____ g

| 2,000.0

---

9. To change grams to kilograms, <u>divide</u> the number of grams by <u>1,000</u> or move the decimal three places to the <u>left</u>.

    Thus:
    1,000.0 g ÷ 1,000 = 1.0 kg or
    1,000.0 g = 1 000.0 = 1.0 kg

    4,000.0 g = _____ kg | 4.0

10. 60.0 g = 0.06 kg

    75.0 g = _____ kg | 0.075

11. 750.0 g = _____ kg | 0.75

12. 3.5 kg = _____ g | 3500

13. 1800 g = _____ kg | 1.8

14. 0.5 kg = _____ g | 500

15. 750 g = _____ kg | 0.75

---

16. The prefix <u>milli</u> indicates one one-thousandth of the unit. A milligram

(mg) is _____ g.

one one-thousandth

---

17. One one-thousandth gram may also

be written _____ g.

0.001

---

18. 4.0 mg = 0.004 g

13.0 mg = _____ g

0.013

---

19. 230.0 mg = _____ g

0.23

---

20. To change grams to milligrams, <u>multiply</u> the number of grams by 1,000 or move the decimal three places to the <u>right</u>.

3.0 g × 1,000 = 3,000.0 mg or
3.0 g = 3,000 = 3,000.0 mg

2.0 g = _____ mg

2,000.0

---

21.   15.0 g = 15,000.0 mg

35.0 g = _____ mg   35,000.0

---

22.   1.5 g = _____ mg   1,500.0

---

23.   To change milligrams to grams,
divide the number of milligrams by
1,000 or move the decimal three
places to the left.

Thus:
1,200.0 mg ÷ 1,000 = 1.2 g or
1,200.0 mg = 1 200.0 = 1.2 g

50.0 mg = _____ g   0.05

---

24.   14.0 mg = 0.014 g

100.0 mg = _____ g   0.10

---

25.   250.0 mg = _____ g   0.25

---

26.   8.0 mg = _____ g   0.008

---

27. 750.0 mg = _____ g

0.75

28. 10.0 g = _____ mg

10,000.0

29. 3.0 g = _____ mg

3,000.0

30. Volume in the metric system is
     expressed in terms of the <u>liter</u>. The

     _____ is the unit of
     volume in the metric system.

liter

31. The <u>liter</u> and the <u>milliliter</u> (ml) are
     most frequently used. You will
     recall that the prefix <u>milli</u> means
     one one-thousandth of a unit.
     Here the prefix <u>milli</u> indicates

     _____ _____

     of a liter.

one one-thousandth

32. One <u>milliliter</u> (ml) and one <u>cubic</u>
     <u>centimeter</u> (cc) are considered
     equivalent.

     Therefore, 10.0 ml and _____
     cc can be used interchangeably.

10.0

---

33. To change liters to milliliters (ml)
<u>multiply</u> the number of liters by
<u>1,000</u> or move the decimal three
places to the <u>right</u>.

Thus:
2.0 liters × 1,000 = 2,000.0 ml (or cc)
or
2.0 liters = 2.000 = 2,000.0 ml (or cc)

10.0 liters = _____ ml (or cc)   10,000.0

---

34. 15.0 liters = 15,000.0 ml (or cc)

33.0 liters = _____ ml   33,000.0
(or cc)

---

35. 4.0 liters = _____ ml   4,000.0
(or cc)

---

36. To change milliliters (or cubic
centimeters) to liters, <u>divide</u> the
number of milliliters by <u>1,000</u> or
move the decimal three places to
the <u>left</u>.

Thus:
1,500.0 ml ÷ 1,000 = 1.5 liters or
1,500.0 ml = 1 500.0 = 1.5 liters

15.0 cc = _____ liters   0.015

---

37. 18.0 cc = 0.018 liters

     250.0 cc = _____ liters   0.25

38. 965.0 cc = _____ liters   0.965

39. 0.25 liters = _____ ml   250.0

40. 4.0 liters = _____ ml   4,000.0

41. 500.0 ml = _____ liters   0.5

42. 1,320.0 ml = _____ liters   1.32

43. 154.0 cc = _____ liters   0.154

44. 1.75 liters = _____ cc   1,750.0

3

Using Household Measurements

Household measurements are those commonly used in everyday home situations. You will recognize these measurements as those used in recipes and on supermarket items. Household measurements are not as accurate as those of the metric and the apothecaries' systems and, therefore, are not used to pour medications when either of the other systems is available. If you examine spoons, cups, and glasses in your own home, it will be evident to you that there is considerable variation in capacity. It may be that the household measurement is the only one you have available when working in a home situation or that it is the easiest system to use in patient teaching. These household measurements are familiar to the patient, and there are situations in which the measurements can be used with safety, such as "normal saline solution" for a gargle.

1. Household <u>measurements</u> are not as accurate as metric or apothecaries' system measurements and therefore are not used as frequently in medicine. However, the home-care nurse often will find accurate measures not available and must use what is available.

Household measures are not as desirable as metric or apothecaries' measures because they are less

_____.   accurate

---

2. <u>Sixty drops</u> (gtt) are considered <u>one teaspoonful</u> (t).

60 gtt (drops) = 1 t (teaspoonful).

Therefore, 120 gtt = _____ t   2

---

3. 5 t = 300 gtt

3 t = _____ gtt   180

---

4. 30 gtt = _____ t $\dfrac{1}{2}$

---

5. 4 t = _____ gtt   240

---

6. 240 gtt = _____ t

4

---

7. 90 gtt = _____t

$1\frac{1}{2}$

---

8. 2 t = _____ gtt

120

---

9. <u>Three</u> <u>teaspoonfuls</u> (t) equal <u>one</u> <u>tablespoonful</u> (T).

3 t (teaspoonfuls) = 1 T (tablespoonful)

9 t = _____ T

3

---

10. 6 T = 18 t

4 T = _____ t

12

---

11. 6 t = _____ T

2

---

12. 3 T = _____ t

9

---

13. 9 t = _____ T

3

---

14. 2 T = _____ t

6

---

15. <u>Two</u> <u>tablespoonfuls</u> (T) equal <u>one</u>
<u>fluid</u> <u>ounce</u>.

2 T = 1 ounce (the word fluid is
usually omitted)

4 T = _____ ounces

2

---

16. 5 ounces = 10 T

4 ounces = _____ T

8

---

17. 12 T = _____ ounces

6

---

18. 3 T = _____ ounces

$1\frac{1}{2}$

---

19. 6 ounces = _____ T

12

---

20. 12 T = _____ ounces

6

---

21. 2 ounces = _____ T

4

22. Eight fluid ounces equal one cupful.

8 ounces = 1 cupful

16 ounces = _____ cupfuls.

2

23. 10 cupfuls = 80 ounces.

3 cupfuls = _____ ounces.

24

24. 48 ounces = _____ cupfuls

6

25. 12 ounces = _____ cupfuls

$1\frac{1}{2}$

26. 3 cupfuls = _____ ounces

24

27. 6 cupfuls = _____ ounces

48

28. 48 ounces = _____ cupfuls

6

29. <u>Two</u> <u>pints</u> (pt) equal <u>one</u> <u>quart</u> (qt).

2 pt (pints) = 1 qt (quart)

Therefore, 4 pt = _____ qt | 2

---

30. 5 qt = 10 pt

3 qt = _____ pt | 6

---

31. 10 qt = _____ pt | 20

---

32. 4 quarts = _____ pints | 8

---

33. 12 pints = _____ quarts | 6

---

34. 2 quarts = _____ pints | 4

---

35. 1 pint = _____ quart(s) | $\dfrac{1}{2}$

Mastering Equivalents

By definition, an equivalent is a given quantity that is considered to be of equal value to a quantity expressed in a different system. In comparing the metric, the apothecaries', and the household systems, a unit of one system never exactly equals a unit of another system. For example, while 1 ounce is exactly 29.5729 grams, in working dosage problems, you will round off to the nearest whole number. Hence, 30 grams is the approximate equivalent of 1 ounce.

By using the approximate equivalent in computation, you will obtain a slightly different answer than if you used the exact equivalent; however, a difference of 10% or less is considered legitimate.

Because these three systems of weights and measures are currently used in the United States, it is most important that you thoroughly understand each of the systems and be able to convert from one to another accurately and without hesitation.

1. There will be times when the three
   measurement systems will have to
   be used <u>interchangeably.</u> The order
   for the drug may be in metric terms,
   and the method of measurement

   available in _____ or

   _____ systems.

   apothecaries'

   household

2. An equivalent is an amount in one
   system that may be substituted for a
   like amount in another system.

   However, the _____ may
   not be exactly equal to the original
   measure.

   equivalent

3. For example, 1.0 g is exactly equal
   to 15.432 grains. In computing
   dosages of medications, however,
   you will substitute 15 grains for 1.0
   grams when necessary.

   We can say that grains 15 is the

   _____ of 1.0 grams.

   equivalent

----

4. When it is necessary to convert from one system to another, it doesn't matter if the desired dose or the on-hand dose is the one that is converted. It is simpler to convert the desired dose to that on hand; therefore, in this text we will

    convert the _____   desired

    _____ to the dose on   dose
    hand.

----

5. In computing dosages of medications, 30.0 grams is considered the equivalent of one ounce (ℨi).

    Therefore, we can say _____ g is   30.0
    ℨi.

----

6. To change <u>grams</u> to <u>ounces</u>, divide the number of grams by 30.

    grams ÷ 30 = _____   ounces

----

7. Example:
   In 60.0 grams there are how many
   ounces?

   grams ÷ 30 = ounces

   60.0 g ÷ 30 = _____ ounces   2

---

8. Example:
   How many ounces are in 150.0
   grams?

   150.0 g ÷ 30 = _____ ounces   5

---

9. How many ounces are in 30 grams?

   30 g ÷ 30 = _____ ounces   1

---

10. How many ounces are in 135
    grams?

    135 g ÷ 30 = _____ ounces $4\frac{1}{2}$

---

11. To change <u>ounces</u> to <u>grams</u>,
    multiply the number of ounces by
    30.

    ounces × 30 = _____   grams

12. Example:
How many grams are in 4 ounces?

ounces × 30 = grams

$4 \times 30 =$ _____   120.0

13. Example:
How many grams are in $6\frac{1}{2}$ ounces?

$6\frac{1}{2} \times 30 =$ _____   195.0

14. How many grams are in 3 ounces?

$3 \times 30 =$ _____   90.0

15. How many grams are in 20 ounces?

$20 \times 30 =$ _____   600.0

16. 40.0 g = ℥ _____ $1\frac{1}{3}$

17. 70.0 g = ℥ _____ $2\frac{1}{3}$

----

18. ʒ8 = _____ g | 240

----

19. ʒ10 = _____ g | 300

----

20. ʒ61 = _____ g | 1,830

----

21. 30.0 cc is considered the equivalent of 1 ounce. In converting from metric to apothecaries' systems you

should consider _____ cc as being equal to ʒi. | 30.0

----

22. To change <u>cc</u> to <u>ounces</u>, divide the number of cc by 30.

cc ÷ 30 = _____ | ounces

----

23. Example:
240.0 cc is how many ounces?

cc ÷ 30 = ounces

240.0 cc ÷ 30 = ʒ _____ | 8

----

24. Example:
How many ounces are there in
180.0 cc?

180.0 cc ÷ 30 = ℥ _____   6

---

25. How many ounces are in 60.0 cc?

60.0 cc ÷ 30 = ℥ _____   2

---

26. How many ounces are in 1,000.0 cc?

1,000.0 cc ÷ 30 = ℥ _____ $33\frac{1}{3}$

---

27. To change <u>ounces</u> to <u>cc</u> multiply the
number of ounces by 30.

ounces × 30 = _____   cc

---

28. Example:
A four-ounce bottle holds how
many cc?

ounces × 30 = cc

℥4 × 30 = _____ cc   120.0

29. Example:
How many cc are in 10 ounces?

℥10 × 30 = _____ cc

300.0

30. How many cc are in 6 ounces?

℥6 × 30 = _____ cc

180.0

31. How many cc are in $2\frac{1}{2}$ ounces?

$℥2\frac{1}{2}$ = _____ cc

75.0

32. 15.0 cc = ℥ _____

$\frac{1}{2}$

33. 10.5 cc = ℥ _____

$3\frac{1}{2}$

34. ℥30 = _____ cc

900

35. $℥4\frac{1}{2}$ = _____ cc

135

---

36. 5 cc = _____ ℨ

0.167

---

37. ℨ15 = _____ cc

0.5

---

38. In computing dosages for some
medications, weight in kilograms is
used. A kilogram is equivalent to
2.2 pounds. Therefore, we can say
2.2 pounds is equivalent to

_____ kilogram (kg).

1

---

39. To change <u>pounds</u> to <u>kilograms</u>,
divide the number of pounds by 2.2.

pounds ÷ 2.2 = _____

kilograms

---

40. Example:
How many kilograms are in 220
pounds?

pounds ÷ 2.2 = kg

220 pounds ÷ 2.2 = _____ kg

100.0

---

41. Example:
How many kilograms are in
15 pounds?

15 pounds ÷ 2.2 = _____ kg   6.8

---

42. How many kilograms are in
44 pounds?

44 pounds ÷ 2.2 = _____ kg   20

---

43. How many kilograms are in
198 pounds?

198 pounds ÷ 2.2 = _____kg   90

---

44. To change <u>kilograms</u> to <u>pounds</u>,
multiply the number of kilograms
by 2.2.

kilograms × 2.2 = _____   pounds

---

45. Example:
How many pounds are equivalent
to 60 kilograms?

kilograms × 2.2 = pounds

60 kg × 2.2 = _____ pounds   132

46. Example:
How many pounds are equivalent
to 20 kilograms?

20 kg × 2.2 = _____ pounds

44

---

47. How many pounds are equivalent
to 500 kilograms?

500 kg × 2.2 = _____ pounds

1100

---

48. How many pounds are equivalent
to 9 kilograms?

9 kg × 2.2 = _____ pounds

19.8

---

49. 132 pounds = _____ kg

60

---

50. 72 kg = _____ pounds

158.4

---

51. 78 kg = _____ pounds

171.6

---

52. 30 kg = _____ pounds

66

53. 84 pounds = _____ kg

38.18

---

54. 100 pounds = _____ kg

45.45

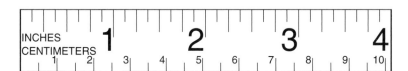

55. The metric equivalent of 1 inch is 2.54 cm. To change <u>inches</u> to <u>cm</u>,

multiply by _____.

2.54

---

56. To change <u>cm</u> to <u>inches</u>, you must

_____ by 2.54.

divide

---

57. How many cm is $3\frac{1}{2}$ inches?

$3\frac{1}{2} \times 2.54 =$ _____

8.89 cm

---

58. How many cm is $\frac{1}{2}$ inch?

$\frac{1}{2} \times 2.54 =$ _____

1.27 cm

59. How many inches is 3 cm?

3 ÷ 2.54 = _____   1.18 inches

60. How many inches is 12 cm?

12 ÷ 2.54 = _____   4.72 inches

61. 3.25 inches = _____ cm   8.26

62. 16 inches = _____ cm   40.64

63. 21 cm = _____ inches   8.27

64. 1 cm = _____ inches   0.39

65. It may be necessary to change a temperature from Celsius (°C) scale to Fahrenheit (°F) scale. To convert a Celsius (°C) reading to Fahrenheit (°F), use the formula:

$$°F = \frac{9}{5} °C + 32°$$

If the °C reading is 37°, the °F is

$$\frac{9}{5}(37°) + 32° = \underline{\hspace{3cm}}.$$

98.6°F

---

66. A Celsius temperature of 50° is

_____°F.

122

---

67. To change a temperature from Fahrenheit (°F) to Celsius (°C), use the formula:

$$°C = \frac{5}{9}(°F - 32°)$$

If the temperature is 100°F, the °C temperature is

$$\frac{5}{9}(100° - 32°) = \underline{\hspace{3cm}}.$$

38°C

---

68. A temperature of 160° F would be

_____°C.

71.1

---

69. 94°F = _____°C | 34.4

---

70. 72°C = _____°F | 161.6

---

71. 57°C = _____°F | 134.6

---

72. 20°F = _____°C | −6.7

---

73. 98.6°F = _____°C | 37

Reading Drug Labels

It is important when dispensing medications to **carefully** read and understand the drug label. Drugs are packaged in several forms: multidose packages and unit dose packages (one dose per package).

Two names generally appear on the label: the trade name and the generic name. The trade name is that name given to the drug by the pharmaceutical company that produces it. The generic name is the general name of a drug with a certain chemical composition. Drugs can be referred to by either the trade name or the generic name.

The label of the drug and the written order must be compared and determined to be a match before the drug is dispensed to the patient.

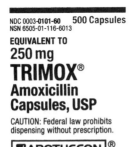
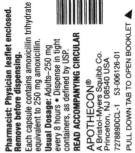

(Courtesy of Bristol-Myers Squibb Company. Used with permission.)

1. Drugs are packaged in several ways.

   These include _____

   and _____.

multiple dose;

unit dose

---

2. The following are drawings of unit dose packages:

pull open	peel open
Capsule	Aspirin 325 mg

| p u l l | Spansule | p e e l | Tablet |

(Borrowed with permission from Henke G. Med-Math: Dosage Calculation, Preparation, and Administration, 3rd ed. Philadelphia: 1999:49.)

   In each package, there is

   _____ dose.

one

----

3. The following is an example of a label on a multiple dose package:

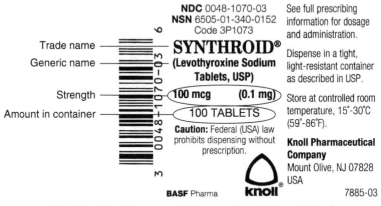

(Courtesy of Knoll Pharmaceutical Company. Used with permission.)

Each multiple dose container contains _____ doses. The important information on the drug label is circled and labeled.	many

----

4. Drugs are labeled with the _____ name and the	generic;
_____ name.	trade

----

5. The trade name has an ® after it. The trade name of the drug is _____.	Synthroid

----

6. Also written on the label is the generic name. The generic name of

the drug is _____.

Levothyroine sodium

7. The strength of the drug is _____ mg.

0.1

8. Read the following label:

(Copyright Eli Lilly and Company. Used with permission.)

The trade name is _____.

Keflex

9. The generic name is

_____.

Cephalexin

10. The strength is _____.

250 mg

---

11. Read the following label:

Sample—For educational use only

Lederle

NDC 0005-3898-46

6505-01-310-4161

SUPRAX®

cefixime

for Oral Suspension
100 mg per 5 mL

Contains 2 g cefixime
as the trihydrate.
Each teaspoonful
(5 mL) contains
100 mg cefixime
when dispensed
as directed.
USUAL DOSAGE:
See accompanying
literature.
CAUTION: Federal law
prohibits dispensing
without prescription.

100 mL
(when reconstituted)

AUG 98

Exp. Date

STORE DRY POWDER AT CONTROLLED
ROOM TEMPERATURE 15-30°C (59-86°F).

4 6505-3898-46 Z3

TO THE PHARMACIST   IMPORTANT
Use this bottle for dispensing.
REMOVE THIS PORTION OF LABEL ONLY
To reconstitute, suspend with **69 mL water.**
Method: Tap the bottle several times to loosen
powder contents prior to reconstitution. Add
approximately half the total amount
of water for reconstitution and shake
well. Add the remainder of water and
shake well.   30241-93   SM3   ©1992

Advantus™
Pharmaceuticals

Marketed by
ADVANTUS
Pharmaceuticals

Lederle

LEDERLE LABORATORIES
DIVISION
American Cyanamid Company
Pearl River, NY 10965

Under License of
Fujisawa Pharmaceutical Co., Ltd.
Osaka, Japan

(Courtesy of Lederle Pharmaceutical Division of American Cyanamid Company. Used with permission.)

The generic name of the drug is _____.	cefixime
12. The trade name of the drug is _____.	Suprax
13. The strength of the drug is _____.	100 mg per 5 ml
14. The bottle contains _____ ml.	100

Calculating Oral Medication Dosage

The most common method of administering medications is by mouth. This is considered the safest method and is usually the easiest for the patient. Medications that are given p.o. (Latin *per os*—by mouth) come in varied forms: pills, tablets, capsules, powders, and liquids.

The dose of medication that is available is frequently different from the dose to be given. Therefore, it is necessary to calculate how many or what part of the oral medication must be given in order to administer the correct dose. Many tablets are scored so that they can be easily broken into halves or quarters. Medications that are soluble in water may be dissolved to divide the dose.

1. In preparing to administer oral medications, you may find that the prescribed dose is different from what is available. When the size of

   the prescribed _____ and that of the medication on hand are not the same, you must determine how much of the available medication should be given.

dose

2. If the size of the tablet on hand is larger than the prescribed dose, less

   than one _____ will be needed.

tablet

3. If the size of the tablet on hand is smaller than the prescribed dose,

   _____ than one tablet will be used.

more

4. To calculate the part of a tablet to

   be used or the _____

   _____ _____, you should use the formula given in frame 5.

number

of tablets

5. Formula:

$$\frac{\text{Desired dose}}{\text{On-hand dose}} \quad \text{or} \quad \frac{D}{H}$$

The desired dose (D) is the

_____ of medication
prescribed.

amount or quantity

---

6. To solve the formula $\frac{D}{H}$ the

quantity D is _____ by   divided
the quantity H.

---

7. Example:
The order is for 10 mg of glipizide
(Glucatrol).

On hand is:
glipizide (Glucatrol) 5 mg.

How many of the tablet(s) would
you use?

Use the formula $\frac{D}{H}$ and substitute

known values: $\dfrac{\underline{\ \ }\text{mg}}{\underline{\ \ }\text{mg}}$ $\dfrac{10\ \text{mg}}{5\ \text{mg}}$

---

8. $\dfrac{D}{H} = \dfrac{10\ \text{mg}}{5\ \text{mg}} = 10\ \text{mg} \div 5\ \text{mg} =$

_____ of the 5 mg tablets will   2
be used.

9. Another way to solve the formula
$\dfrac{D}{H}$ is to reduce the fraction to its
lowest terms:

$$\frac{D}{H} = \frac{500 \text{ mg}}{250 \text{ mg}} = \frac{\underline{\quad ? \quad}}{\underline{\quad ? \quad}}$$

2 mg
1 mg

---

10. $\dfrac{2}{1} =$ _____ of the 250-mg tablets
will be used.

2

---

11. You should use the method that
you find easiest, or use the two

_____ interchangeably.

methods

---

12. Example:
The order is for furosemide (Lasix)
20 mg.

On hand is:
furosemide (Lasix)
40 mg tablet.

$$\frac{D}{H} = \frac{\underline{\quad ? \quad} \text{ mg}}{\underline{\quad ? \quad} \text{ mg}}$$

20
40

Substitute the known values.

13. $\dfrac{D}{H} = \dfrac{20 \text{ mg}}{40 \text{ mg}} = \dfrac{1}{2}$

    or _____ tablet of furosemide
(Lasix) 40 mg will be used.

$\dfrac{1}{2}$

---

14. Using the alternative method:

$\dfrac{D}{H} = \dfrac{20 \text{ mg}}{40 \text{ mg}} = 20 \text{ mg} \div 40 \text{ mg} =$

_____ tablet(s) of furosemide
(Lasix) 40 mg will be used.

$\dfrac{1}{2}$

---

15. The order is for phenobarbital
60 mg.

    On hand is:

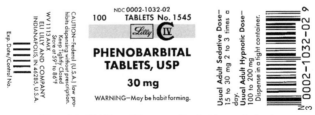

(Copyright Eli Lilly and Company. Used with permission.)

$\dfrac{D}{H} = \dfrac{\_\_?\_\_ \text{ mg}}{\_\_?\_\_ \text{ mg}}$
(Substitute the known values)

60
30

---

16. $\dfrac{D}{H} = \dfrac{60 \text{ mg}}{30 \text{ mg}} = 2$

or _____ tablet(s) of
phenobarbital 30 mg will be used.

2

---

17. From the following container give
15 mg of phenobarbital.

_____

$\dfrac{1}{2}$ tablet

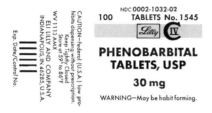
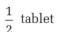

(Copyright Eli Lilly and Company. Used with permission.)

---

18. From dipyridamole (Persantine)
25 mg, give 50 mg.

_____

$\dfrac{D}{H} = \dfrac{50 \text{ mg}}{25 \text{ mg}} = 2$ tablets

---

19. From digoxin (Lanoxin) 0.25 mg,
give 0.125 mg.

$\dfrac{D}{H} = \dfrac{0.125 \text{ mg}}{0.25 \text{ mg}} = \dfrac{1}{2}$ tablet

---

20. From propranolol hydrochloride (Inderal) 10 mg, give 40 mg.

$$\frac{D}{H} = \frac{40 \text{ mg}}{10 \text{ mg}} = 4 \text{ tablets}$$

21. From the following container give 750 mg.

$$\frac{D}{H} = \frac{750 \text{ mg}}{250 \text{ mg}} = 3 \text{ capsules}$$

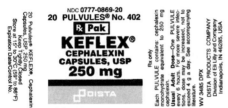

(Copyright Eli Lilly and Company. Used with permission.)

22. When liquids are ordered, use the formula:

$$\frac{\text{Desired dose}}{\text{On-hand dose}} \times \text{Volume or } \frac{D}{H} \times V.$$

The container is labeled according to the amount of the drug in a given volume of the liquid. In this case the amount of drug in a given

volume will be the _____ of the

formula $\frac{D}{H} \times V$.

D

23. This is the label for cefixime
(Suprax):

Sample—For educational use only.

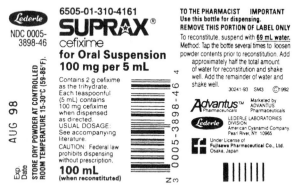

(Courtesy of Lederle Pharmaceutical Division of American Cyanamid Company. Used with permission.)

How will you give 250 mg?

$$\frac{D}{H} \times V = \frac{250 \text{ mg}}{100 \text{ mg}} \times 5 \text{ cc} =$$

_____ cc v.   12.5

---

24. The label indicates that there are
125 mg of amoxicillin (Amox) per
5 cc. How will you give 250 mg?

$$\frac{D}{H} \times V = \frac{250 \text{ mg}}{125 \text{ mg}} \times 5 \text{ cc} =$$

_____ cc will be given.   10

25. From:

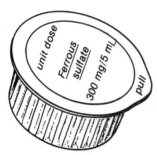

(Borrowed with permission from Henke G. Med-Math: Dosage Calculation, Preparation, and Administration, 3rd ed. Philadelphia: 1999:49.)

Give 450 mg.

$$\frac{D}{H} \times V = \frac{450 \text{ mg}}{300 \text{ mg}} \times 5 \text{ ml} = 7.5 \text{ ml}$$

---

26. From:

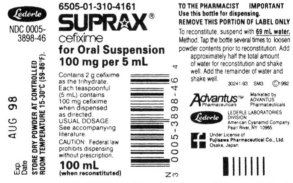

(Courtesy of Lederle Pharmaceutical Division of American Cyanamid Company. Used with permission.)

Give 250 mg.

$$\frac{D}{H} \times V = \frac{250 \text{ mg}}{100 \text{ mg}} \times 5 \text{ ml} = 12.5 \text{ ml}$$

Selecting a Syringe for Parenteral Injections

Many medications are given parenterally, that is, by injection—subcutaneously, intramuscularly, or intradermally. Three types of syringes are used: tuberculin, insulin, and hypodermic. The syringe selected is determined by the route and the amount of drug to be given.

Insulin syringes are especially designed for use with U-100 insulin and are calibrated in 1-unit measures.

The tuberculin syringe is a narrow 1-ml syringe. It is calibrated in $\frac{1}{10}$- and $\frac{1}{100}$-ml units on one side and minims on the other side.

The hypodermic syringe comes in various sizes. The most commonly used size is a 3-ml syringe calibrated in $\frac{1}{10}$-ml increments on one side and minims on the other side.

In this chapter, you will learn which syringe is appropriate to use to administer a given drug.

1. You should select a syringe to use depending on the quantity of solution to be given, the drug, the route, and the body size. To determine which syringe to use, you must calculate the

    _____ of the solution.   quantity

2. The tuberculin syringe is a narrow

    1-ml syringe. It is marked off in

    $\frac{1}{10}$ ml, $\frac{1}{100}$ ml, and minims. The
    tuberculin syringe is used for

    injections _____ than   less
    1 ml.

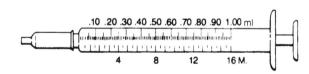

3. The insulin syringe is a narrow 1.0-ml or 0.5-ml syringe marked off in single units. It is used <u>only</u> for insulin that contains 100 units/ml.

    The insulin syringe <u>would</u>/   would not
    <u>would</u> <u>not</u> be used for heparin.

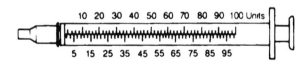

4. The hypodermic syringe most
    commonly used is a 3-ml syringe. It
    is marked off in $\frac{1}{10}$ ml and minims.

    The _____ syringe   hypodermic
    would be used for quantities of
    drug greater than 1 ml.

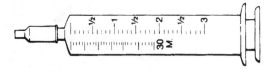

    The hypodermic syringe also comes
    in sizes of 5 ml marked off in $\frac{1}{5}$ ml,
    10 ml marked off in $\frac{1}{5}$ ml, 20 ml
    marked off in 1-ml increments,
    30 ml marked off in increments of
    1 ml, and 50 ml marked off in
    increments of 1 ml.

5. Needle gauges vary. The higher the
    gauge number, the smaller the
    needle. For instance, a 25-gauge

    needle is _____ than a   smaller
    21-gauge needle.

6. The lengths of needles also vary, from $\frac{3}{8}$ inch to $1\frac{1}{2}$ inch. A

25-gauge needle, $\frac{1}{2}$ to $\frac{5}{8}$ inch long, is used for a subcutaneous injection since only the subcutaneous layer is to be penetrated.

To give a subcutaneous injection, the

nurse would use a _____ gauge,   25

_____-inch needle. $\frac{1}{2}$ or $\frac{5}{8}$

7. The tuberculin syringe has a 26- to 27-gauge needle, $\frac{3}{8}$ to $\frac{5}{8}$ inch long, for intradermal injections. The tuberculin syringe with its small needle would be used for

_____ injections. The   intradermal
hypodermic syringe has a needle of 18 to 22 gauge and

is 1 to $1\frac{1}{2}$ inches in length. The needle size to be used is determined by the viscosity of the medication and the size of the patient.

---

8. If a medication for intramuscular injection is drawn up in a tuberculin syringe because it is a quantity less than 1 ml, the needle must be changed. If it is for an intramuscular injection, the needle would be changed to a(n)

_____-gauge,

_____-inch needle.

18- to 22

1 to $1\frac{1}{2}$

---

9. Some medications come in prefilled cartridges that are inserted into special holders in order to be able to inject them. These are called Tubex or Carpuject. If these are used, read the manufacturer's directions.

---

10. Now let's determine which syringe to use for the following orders. Heparin 5,000 units SC is ordered. The vial contains 20,000 units per ml. How much would you need?

$$\frac{D}{H} \times V = \underline{\hspace{3cm}}$$

Fill in the proper numbers and complete the problem.

$$\frac{5,000 \text{ units}}{20,000 \text{ units}} \times 1 \text{ ml} = .25 \text{ ml}$$

---

11. In the preceding problem, a(n)

_____ syringe would be
used. The needle must be changed

tuberculin

to a(n) _____ -gauge,

25

_____ inch needle to
give a subcutaneous injection.

$\dfrac{1}{2}$ or $\dfrac{5}{8}$

12. Mark the point to which the
medicine amount in question 10
should be drawn up to in the
syringe:

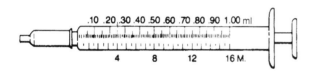

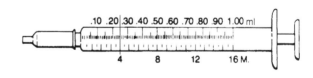

13. The order reads 25 units Humulin
N insulin SC in A.M. The vial
contains Humulin N 100 units/ml.

A(n) _____ syringe would

insulin

be used and _____ units
of insulin drawn into the syringe.

25

----

14. Hydroxyzine 75 mg IM is ordered. The vial reads 100 mg/2 ml. A(n)

_____ syringe would be used and

3-ml hypodermic

_____ ml drawn into the syringe.

1.5

----

15. Meperidine 25 mg IM is ordered. You have the following vial:

Meperidine HCl ⓊⒸ
Injection, USP
Warning: May be habit forming
50 mg/mL
071156R02 **For IM, SC or Slow IV* Use**
*See Insert
30 mL Multiple Dose Vial
Caution: Federal law prohibits
dispensing without prescription.
ASTRA®
Astra Pharmaceutical Products, Inc.
Westborough, MA 01581

NDC 0186-1284-01
Each mL contains:
50 mg meperidine HCl
(Warning: May be habit forming), 1 mg metacresol as the
preservative, and sodium hydroxide and/or hydrochloric
acid to adjust pH 3.5–6.0.
See insert for dosage and
full prescribing information.
DO NOT USE IF SOLUTION
IS DISCOLORED OR
CONTAINS A PRECIPITATE.
Store at controlled
room temperature
15°–30°C (59°–86°F).

APPROXIMATE VOLUME (mL)
25
20
15
10
5

(Reproduced with permission of Astra Pharmaceuticals, L.P., 50 Otis St., Westborough, MA 01581-4500.)

a(n) _____ syringe with needle changed to

tuberculin 18- to 22-

_____ gauge would be

1 to $1\frac{1}{2}$ inches long

used and _____ ml given.

.50

----

16. The order reads: "Meperidine 75 mg IM." The vial contains 100 mg/ml. What syringe and needle would be used and how much medicine given?

Use a tuberculin syringe and change the needle to an 18- to 22-gauge needle, 1 to $1\frac{1}{2}$ inches long

$$\frac{D}{H} \times V = \frac{75 \text{ mg}}{100 \text{ mg}} \times 1 \text{ ml} = \frac{3}{4} \times 1 \text{ ml} = \frac{3}{4} \text{ ml}$$

17. The order reads "Atropine sulfate 0.4 mg IM." The vial contains 1 mg/ml. What syringe and needle would be used and how much medicine given?

Use a tuberculin syringe and change the needle to an 18- to 22-gauge needle, 1 to $1\frac{1}{2}$ inches long

$$\frac{D}{H} \times V = \frac{0.4 \text{ mg}}{1 \text{ mg}} \times 1 \text{ ml} = 0.4 \text{ ml}$$

18. The order reads hydroxyzine hydrochloride 50 mg. The vial contains 50 mg/ml. What syringe and needle would be used and how much medicine given?

Use a 3-ml hypodermic syringe with an 18- to 22-gauge needle, 1 to $1\frac{1}{2}$ inches long

$$\frac{D}{H} \times V = \frac{50 \text{ mg}}{50 \text{ mg}} \times 1 \text{ ml} = 1 \text{ ml}$$

19. The order reads: "Humulin regular insulin 20 units SC." On hand is a vial with Humulin regular 100 units/ml. What syringe would be used and how much medicine given?

Use an insulin syringe and draw 20 units of insulin

20. The order reads: "Cimetidine 300 mg IM." The drug comes 300 mg/2 ml. What syringe would be used and how much medicine given?

Use a 3-ml hypodermic syringe and draw 2 ml of medication

8

Calculating Injectable Liquid Dosage

There are many drugs that can be stored safely in liquid form. These drugs are packaged in ampules (single-dose) or vials (single-dose or multiple-dose) and are labeled according to the amount of the drug in the ampule or in a fractional part of the vial; for example, meperidine hydrochloride 50 mg (ampule), or meperidine hydrochloride 50 mg/cc (multi-dose vial). These drugs are administered parenterally.

Should the order for the medication and the drug that is available differ in dosage, you will use the formula discussed in this chapter to determine the quantity of solution to be given. Remember, as in working all dosage problems, two systems of weights and measures cannot be used in one problem without first converting the units to a common system.

1. Drugs for hypodermic injection are often kept in solutions of various strengths. These drugs are packaged in <u>ampules</u> or <u>vials</u>. An ampule holds a single dose, while a vial holds more than one dose. If you have four doses packaged together in one container, this container is

    called a _____.

    vial

2. The container will be labeled with the <u>amount of drug</u> in the ampule or the fractional part of the vial. A vial labeled gr $\frac{1}{4}$ per cc would contain gr $\frac{1}{4}$ of the drug in each

    _____ of solution.

    cc

3. When the prescribed dose and the label on the ampule are the same, you should withdraw

    _____ of the solution in the ampule.

    all

4. You are to give 50.0 mg of a drug in a vial labeled 50.0 mg per cc. You

should withdraw _____ cc of solution from the vial.

1.0

---

5. When the prescribed dose differs from the label, you must determine

how much of the _____ must be used to give the prescribed dose.

solution

---

6. To determine the amount of solution required, use the following formula:

$$\frac{D}{H} \times V = x$$

In this formula:

D stands for _____ .

desired dose

H stands for _____ .

dose on hand

V stands for the volume on hand
x stands for the desired volume.

7. Example:
    The vial is labeled "Ceftriaxone
    1 gm/4 ml."

    Give 125 mg.

    $$\frac{D}{H} \times V = x$$

    $$\frac{125 \text{ mg}}{1000 \text{ mg}} \times 4 \text{ ml} = x$$

    $0.125 \times 4 \text{ ml} = x$

    $x =$ _____

    _____

    0.5 ml of the ceftriaxone
    will be given

8. Example:
    The vial is labeled
    "Prochlorperazine:
    5.0 mg per ml."

    How would you give 8.0 mg of the
    drug?

    $$\frac{D}{H} \times V = x$$

    $$\frac{8.0 \text{ mg}}{?} \times \underline{\quad ? \quad} = x$$

    5.0 mg   1.0 ml

9. $\dfrac{8.0 \text{ mg}}{5.0 \text{ mg}} \times 1.0 \text{ ml} =$

Finish the calculation and label the answer.

$1.6 \times 1 \text{ ml} = 1.6 \text{ ml of}$
prochlorperazine will be
needed to give 8.0 mg

---

10. From a streptomycin solution containing 500.0 mg in 1.0 ml, give 400.0 mg.

$$\frac{D}{H} \times V = x$$

$$\frac{4\cancel{0}\cancel{0}.\cancel{0} \text{ mg}}{5\cancel{0}\cancel{0}.\cancel{0} \text{ mg}} \times 1 \text{ ml} = x$$

$0.8 \times 1.0 \text{ ml} = x$
$x = 0.8 \text{ ml of the}$
streptomycin solution in
1.0 ml is needed to give
streptomycin 400.0 mg

---

11. From a medication from the following vial, give 75.0 mg of the meperdine.

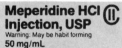

Meperidine HCl
Injection, USP
Warning: May be habit forming
50 mg/mL
071156/02 **For IM, SC or Slow IV* Use**
*See Insert
30 mL Multiple Dose Vial
Caution: Federal law prohibits
dispensing without prescription.
ASTRA®
Astra Pharmaceutical Products, Inc.
Westborough, MA 01581

NDC 0186-1284-01
Each mL contains
50 mg meperidine HCl
(Warning: May be habit forming), 1 mg metacresol as the
preservative, and sodium hydroxide and/or hydrochloric
acid to adjust pH 3.5–6.0.
See insert for dosage and
full prescribing information.
DO NOT USE IF SOLUTION
IS DISCOLORED OR
CONTAINS A PRECIPITATE.
Store at controlled
room temperature
15°–30°C (59°–86°F).

(Reproduced with permission of Astra Pharmaceuticals, L.P.,
50 Otis St., Westborough, MA 01581-4500.)

$$\frac{D}{H} \times V = x$$

$$\frac{75.\cancel{0} \text{ mg}}{50.\cancel{0} \text{ mg}} \times 1 \text{ ml} = x$$

$1.5 \times 1.0 \text{ ml} = x$
$x = 1.5 \text{ ml of meperdine}$
solution 50.0 mg per 1 ml
will be used to give
meperdine 75.0 mg

12. Give chlorpromazine 0.050 g from a
    solution labeled 25.0 mg per ml.

$$0.050 \text{ g} = 50.0 \text{ mg}$$

$$\frac{D}{H} \times V = x$$

$$\frac{50.\cancel{0} \text{ mg}}{25.\cancel{0} \text{ mg}} \times 1.0 \text{ ml} = x$$

$$2 \times 1.0 \text{ ml} = x$$

$$x = 2.0 \text{ ml of}$$

chlorpromazine solution
labeled 25.0 mg/ml is
needed to give 0.050 g

---

13. From hydroxyzine 100 mg per 2 ml,
    give 75 mg.

$$\frac{D}{H} \times V = x$$

$$\frac{75 \text{ mg}}{100 \text{ mg}} \times 2 \text{ ml} = x$$

$$0.75 \times 2 \text{ ml} = x$$

$$x = 1.5 \text{ ml of hydroxyzine}$$

solution of 100 mg per
2 ml is required to give
75 mg

---

14. From digitoxin 0.2 mg/ml, give
    0.3 mg.

$$\frac{D}{H} \times V = x$$

$$\frac{0.3 \text{ mg}}{0.2 \text{ mg}} \times 1.0 \text{ ml} = x$$

$$1.5 \times 1.0 \text{ ml} = x$$

$$x = 1.5 \text{ ml of digitoxin}$$

0.2 mg/ml equals 0.3 mg

Administering Drugs Measured in Units

The strength of certain medications is measured in units. A unit is a specifically defined amount of anything subject to measurement. The unit is defined for each drug and there is *no relationship* between the strength of a unit of one drug and a unit of another drug. A unit of heparin cannot be compared to a unit of penicillin. It is also important to note that cubic centimeters and units are not interchangeable.

Insulin is an example of a medication that is measured in units. It is supplied in vials with 100 units per ml. The least complicated and most accurate way to measure insulin is to use an insulin syringe. This is a special 1.0-ml syringe calibrated to measure units rather than cubic centimeters and minims.

When you do not have an insulin syringe to give insulin, you can measure the dose by using a tuberculin syringe or an ordinary 3.0-ml hypodermic syringe. The quantity of insulin to be given is calculated by using the formula presented in this chapter and is measured in minims or cubic centimeters.

The formula (which is the same basic formula you have used before) can be used to calculate the dose of any drug that is measured in units.

1. Many biologicals are supplied in vials containing a <u>specified</u> <u>number</u> <u>of</u> <u>units</u> <u>per</u> <u>cubic</u> <u>centimeter</u> of the solution. A vial labeled 1,500 units per cc would contain

   _____ units of the drug in each cc of the solution.

   1,500

2. The potency of the unit of each product is defined by the United States Pharmacopeia. The unit may also be called a U.S.P.

   _____.

   unit

3. These drugs are ordered according

   to the number of _____ to be given.

   units

4. When the vial is labeled 1,500 U.S.P. units (or 1,500 units) per cc,

   _____ cc of solution will be withdrawn to give 1,500 units.

   1.0

5. When the prescribed dose differs
    from what is on hand, the correct
    dose must be calculated as to how

    much of the _____ must   solution
    be given.

---

6. Again use the basic formula:

    $$\frac{\text{Desired dose}}{\text{On-hand dose}} \; \frac{(D)}{(H)} \times V \left(\text{Volume}\right)$$

    Example:
    The order is for 4,500 units of
    tetanus antitoxin. The label on
    the vial is "Tetanus Antitoxin:
    1,500 units per milliliter." How
    much solution will be needed?

    We will work together step by step:

    $$\frac{D}{H} \times V = \frac{4,500 \text{ units}}{?} \times 1 \text{ ml}$$ 1,500 units

---

7. $$\frac{D}{H} \times V = \frac{4,500 \text{ ml}}{1,500 \text{ units per ml}} \times 1 \text{ ml}$$

    $$\frac{45}{15} \times 1 \text{ ml} = \underline{\hspace{3cm}}$$ 3.0 ml

    of tetanus antitoxin solution
    containing 1,500 units per ml will
    be needed to give 4,500 units of
    tetanus antitoxin.

8. Example:
Using a penicillin solution containing 100,000 units in 1.0 cc, give 40,000 units of the drug.

$$\frac{D}{H} \times V = \underline{\hspace{3cm}}$$

Substitute values and complete calculations. Label answer.

$$\frac{40,000 \text{ units}}{100,000 \text{ units}} \times 1 \text{ cc} =$$

$$\frac{4}{10} \times 1 \text{ cc} = 0.4 \text{ cc}$$

of penicillin solution containing 100,000 units in 1.0 cc will be needed to give 40,000 units of penicillin

9. Example:
The order is for 25 units of Humulin N insulin. The label on the vial reads: "Humulin N: 100 units/cc."
How many cc are needed?

$$\frac{D}{H} \times V = \underline{\hspace{3cm}}$$

$$\frac{25 \text{ units}}{100 \text{ units}} \times 1 \text{ cc} =$$

$.25 \times 1$ cc $= .25$ cc of Humulin N will be needed to give 25 units

10. Example:
The order is for 7,500 units of
heparin sodium. The label reads:
"Heparin sodium: 5,000 units/ml."
How many ml are needed?

$$\frac{D}{H} \times V = \underline{\hspace{4cm}}$$

$$\frac{7{,}500 \text{ units}}{5{,}000 \text{ units}} \times 1 \text{ ml} =$$

$$\frac{75}{50} \times 1 \text{ ml} = 1.5 \text{ ml}$$

will be needed to give
7,500 units heparin sodium

---

11. From a vial labeled "Heparin
sodium 20,000 units per ml," give
5,000 units.

$$\frac{D}{H} \times V = x$$

$$\frac{5{,}\cancel{000} \text{ units}}{20{,}\cancel{000} \text{ units}} \times 1 \text{ ml} = x$$

$x = 0.25$ ml of heparin
sodium solution containing
20,000 units of heparin is
needed

12. Give 50,000 units of sodium penicillin-G from a vial labeled 1,000,000 units/10 ml.

$$\frac{D}{H} \times V = x$$

$$\frac{5\cancel{0},\cancel{0}\cancel{0}\cancel{0} \text{ units}}{1,00\cancel{0},\cancel{0}\cancel{0}\cancel{0} \text{ units}} \times 10 \text{ ml} = x$$

$$\frac{5}{100} \times 10 \text{ ml} = x$$

$$0.5 \times 10 \text{ ml} = x$$

$x = 0.5$ ml of sodium penicillin G solution containing 1,000,000 units/ 10 ml is needed

13. Give penicillin 600,000 units from a solution labeled 3,000,000 units/ 5.0 ml.

$$\frac{D}{H} \times V = x$$

$$\frac{6\cancel{0}\cancel{0},\cancel{0}\cancel{0}\cancel{0}}{3,00\cancel{0},\cancel{0}\cancel{0}\cancel{0}} \times 5 \text{ ml} = x$$

$$\frac{6}{30} \times 5 \text{ ml} = x$$

$$0.2 \times 5 \text{ ml} = x$$

$x = 1.0$ ml of penicillin labeled 3,000,000 units/ 5 ml is needed

14. How many cc of NPH insulin (100 units/cc) will be needed to give 60 units?

$$\frac{D}{H} \times V = x$$

$$\frac{60 \text{ units}}{100 \text{ units}} \times 1.0 \text{ cc} = x$$

$$\frac{6}{10} \times 1 \text{ cc} = x$$

$$x = 0.6 \text{ cc of NPH insulin is needed}$$

15. From a vial labeled "Heparin sodium 5,000 units per ml," give 3,000 units.

$$\frac{D}{H} \times V = x$$

$$\frac{3,\cancel{000} \text{ units}}{5,\cancel{000} \text{ units}} \times 1 \text{ ml} = x$$

$$\frac{3}{5} \times 1 \text{ ml} = x$$

$$x = 0.6 \text{ ml of heparin sodium labeled 5,000 units per ml will be needed}$$

16. Give 2500 units of heparin from the following vial.

NDC 0002-7217-01
5 mL   VIAL No. 520

**HEPARIN SODIUM
INJECTION, USP
10,000 USP
Units per mL**
Rx only
Multiple Dose
See literature for dosage.
Each mL contains 10,000 USP
Heparin units, derived from por-
cine intestinal mucosa, sodium
chloride 0.1%.
Preservative—1% benzyl alcohol
added during manufacture. Sodi-
um hydroxide and/or hydrochloric
acid may have been added during
manufacture to adjust pH.
Store at 25°C (77°F): (see insert)
Eli Lilly and Company
Indianapolis, IN 46285, USA
● WW 1601 AMX ●
Exp. Date/Control No.

(Copyright Eli Lilly and Company. Used with permission.)

$$\frac{D}{H} \times V = x$$

$$\frac{25\!\!\!/00 \text{ units}}{10,0\!\!\!/00 \text{ units}} \times 1 \text{ ml} = x$$

$$\frac{25}{100} \times 1 \text{ ml} = x$$

$x = 0.25$ ml of heparin
sodium will be needed.

10

Preparing Drugs Packaged as Powders and Tablets

Drugs that are unstable in solution may also be packaged in dry form in ampules or vials. When you are ready to use the drug, it is dissolved in the correct diluent. Information concerning the correct diluent is packaged with the drug or can be obtained from the pharmacist or from pharmacology books. When a multi-dose vial is used, the vial must be relabeled stating the amount of drug contained in each cubic centimeter of the fluid and the date the fluid was prepared.

The formula needed to solve this type of conversion problem is presented here. This formula is used only when the amount of the drug does not increase the amount of the solution. When the drug increases the amount of the solution, specific directions as to the quantity of diluent are packaged with the drug and must be followed explicitly.

1. Certain drugs come from the pharmacy in <u>dry powder form</u> in a vial. The vial may contain the quantity of drug required for a single injection or may contain enough medication for several

    _____ .

doses

---

2. To determine the amount of diluent needed, a proportion must be used.

The proportion formula to determine the amount of diluent needed is:

$$\frac{\text{Desired units}}{\text{On-hand units}} = \frac{\text{Desired volume}}{x \text{ volume}}$$

x volume is the amount of diluent that will be added to the dry drug.

Example:
The label on a vial of powdered penicillin reads: "Penicillin: 1,000,000 U.S.P. units." The order reads penicillin 100,000 units stat and b.i.d. How many cubic centimeters of diluent will be needed to produce a solution containing 100,000 units per cc?

Use the formula above:

$$\frac{DU}{HU} = \frac{V}{x}$$

Substitute values:

$$\frac{100,000 \text{ units}}{1,000,000 \text{ units}} = \frac{?}{x}$$

1.0 cc

3. $\dfrac{100{,}000 \text{ units}}{1{,}000{,}000 \text{ units}} = \dfrac{1.0 \text{ cc}}{x}$

100,000 : 1,000,000 : : 1.0 cc : x

$100{,}000x = 1{,}000{,}000$ cc

$x =$ _____

_____

_____

10.0 cc of diluent will be needed to produce penicillin solution of 100,000 units/cc

4. After the diluent has been added to the vial, the vial must be labeled as to the number of units in each

_____.

cc

5. Another example:
How much diluent will be needed to make a solution of 100,000 units per cc if the vial contains 2,000,000 units of dry drug?

$\dfrac{\text{DU}}{\text{HU}} = \dfrac{V}{x}$

$\dfrac{?}{?} = \dfrac{1.0 \text{ cc}}{x}$

100,000
2,000,000

6. $\dfrac{100,000 \text{ units}}{2,000,000 \text{ units}} = \dfrac{1.0 \text{ cc}}{x}$

$100,000 : 2,000,000 : : 1.0 \text{ cc} : x$

$100,000x = 2,000,000 \text{ cc}$

$x = $ _____

_____

_____

20.0 cc of diluent will be needed to make a solution of 100,000 units/cc

7. Some drugs may increase the volume of the solution. The formula $\dfrac{DU}{HU} = \dfrac{V}{x}$ can be used only when the volume of the dry drug does not increase the volume of the

_____.

solution

8. When the dry drug increases the volume of the solution, specific instructions are given by the manufacturer for the

_____ of diluent to use.

amount

9. Example:
   Streptomycin sulfate for injection. The vial contains 1.0 g of the dry drug. Instructions: for 100 mg per cc, add 9.2 cc of diluent.

   9.2 cc of diluent is added to the dry drug, which gives a total of 10.0 cc of solution, where each cc contains

   _____ of the drug.   100.0 mg

10. How much diluent is required to prepare a solution of benzathine penicillin G of 500,000 units per cc when the vial contains 1,000,000 units of the dry drug?

$$\frac{DU}{HU} = \frac{V}{x}$$

$$\frac{500,000 \text{ units}}{1,000,000 \text{ units}} = \frac{1.0 \text{ cc}}{x}$$

500,000 : 1,000,000 : :
1.0 cc : x
500,000x = 1,000,000 cc
x = 2.0 cc diluent is needed to prepare a solution of benzathine penicillin G 500,000 units per cc

11. Given a vial containing 750 units of a drug in dry form, how will you prepare a solution containing 150 units per cc?

$$\frac{DU}{HU} = \frac{V}{x}$$

$$\frac{150 \text{ units}}{750 \text{ units}} = \frac{1.0 \text{ cc}}{x}$$

$150 : 750 : : 1.0 \text{ cc} : x$

$150x = 750.0 \text{ cc}$

$x = 5.0 \text{ cc}$ diluent is needed to prepare a solution containing 150 units of drug per cc

12. How much diluent is needed to give a solution of 25,000 units per cc if the vial contains 200,000 units of dry drug?

$$\frac{DU}{HU} = \frac{V}{x}$$

$$\frac{25,000 \text{ units}}{200,000 \text{ units}} = \frac{1.0 \text{ cc}}{x}$$

$25,000 : 200,000 : : 1.0 \text{ cc} : x$

$25,000x = 200,000.0 \text{ cc}$

$x = 8.0 \text{ cc}$ diluent is needed to prepare a solution containing 25,000 units of drug per cc

13. A vial of potassium penicillin G contains 2,000,000 units of the dry drug. How much diluent is needed to make a solution that contains 400,000 units per cc?

$$\frac{DU}{HU} = \frac{V}{x}$$

$$\frac{400,000 \; \text{units}}{2,000,000 \; \text{units}} = \frac{1.0 \; cc}{x}$$

400,000 : 2,000,000 : :
1.0 cc : x

$400,000x = 2,000,000.0$ cc

$x = 5.0$ cc diluent is needed to prepare a solution containing 400,000 units of potassium penicillin G per cc

Mixing Parenteral Medications

Often, two drugs are mixed in a syringe to decrease the frequency of injection. The drugs mixed must be compatible; that is, they must not form a precipitate when mixed.

Mixing of drugs is common practice when two types of insulin are ordered or when preoperative medications are ordered.

Always check drug compatibility with the pharmacist or with a drug compatibility chart. If the drugs form a precipitate when mixed, discard the mixed solution and inject each drug separately.

In this chapter, you will learn how to mix two drugs together in a syringe.

1. It is possible to mix more than one medication in the same syringe to inject into the patient. This can provide for patient comfort by <u>decreasing/increasing</u> the number of injections needed.

decreasing

2. The two medications must be checked to see that they are compatible—in other words, that they don't react to form a precipitate. If a precipitate forms,

    you _____ give the injection.

cannot

3. When mixing two medications, it is important to not contaminate the medication left in one vial with the other medication. If contamination occurs, the contaminated drug must

    be _____.

discarded

4. When withdrawing two drugs from
two separate vials, draw air into a
syringe in an amount equal to the
solution being withdrawn into vial

   #1. Inject this air into _____   vial

   _____, being careful to keep the   1
   needle out of the medication.
   Withdraw the needle and syringe
   from vial #1 without the
   medication.

5. Draw air into the syringe equaling
the amount of solution to be
withdrawn from vial #2 and inject

   this air into _____   vial

   _____.   2

6. Withdraw the correct amount of
solution from vial #2. Change the
needle and insert the syringe with
the new needle into vial #1.
Withdraw the correct amount of
solution and remove the needle and
syringe from vial #1. The syringe

   has a _____ of the   mixture
   medications from vials #1 and #2,
   but neither is contaminated.

The technique is demonstrated in
the following diagram:

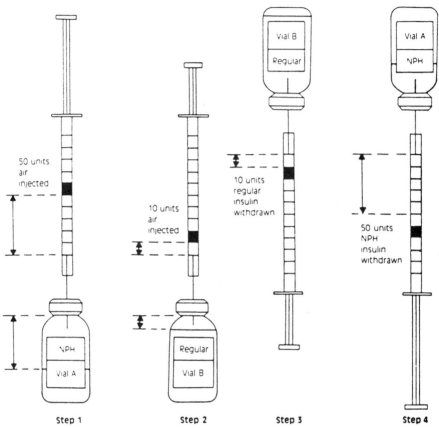

Step 1 Step 2 Step 3 Step 4

(Borrowed with permission from Taylor C, Lillis C, LeMone P. Fundamentals of Nursing: The Art and
Science of Nursing Care. Philadelphia: Lippincott-Raven, 1997:622.)

7. If a multi-dose vial and a single-
   dose vial are used, withdraw the
   medication from the multi-dose vial

   first to prevent _____.   contamination

8. Example:
The order reads: "Meperidine 50 mg IM, hydroxyzine 50 mg IM on call to O.R." Meperidine is packaged in a vial containing 100 mg/cc; hydroxyzine in a vial containing 50 mg/cc.

Fill in the blanks.

You will need _____ cc of meperidine and

_____ cc of

hydroxyzine.

$$\frac{D}{H} \times V = \frac{50 \text{ mg}}{100 \text{ mg}} \times 1 \text{ cc}$$
$$= 0.5 \text{ cc meperidine}$$

$$\frac{D}{H} \times V = \frac{50 \text{ mg}}{50 \text{ mg}} \times 1 \text{ cc}$$
$$= 1 \text{ cc hydroxyzine}$$

9. Use a _____

syringe and draw up _____ cc of air and inject into the meperidine vial.

3-ml hypodermic

0.5

10. _____ the needle and syringe from the meperidine vial.

Remove

11. Draw up 1 cc of air and inject into

the _____ vial.   hydroxyzine
Withdraw 1 cc of the medication
and remove the needle and syringe
from the hydroxyzine vial.

---

12. _____ the needle and   Change
place the needle and syringe into
the meperidine vial.

---

13. Withdraw 0.5 cc of meperidine to a

total of _____ cc in the syringe.   1.5

---

14. Insulins vary in their duration of
action. There are short-acting,
intermediate-acting, and long-acting
insulins. (Review in a
pharmacology text.) Often, two
insulins are ordered together. They
can be mixed in the same

_____ syringe.   insulin

15. If the order reads 10 U regular insulin (short acting) and 25 U NPH (intermediate acting) SC before breakfast, and you have 100 units/cc insulin on hand, these two would be mixed in the following way:	
Draw 25 units of air into the syringe and inject 25 units of air into the	
_____ vial. Withdraw the needle and syringe from the NPH insulin vial.	NPH
16. Draw 10 units of air into the syringe	
and inject into the _____ insulin vial.	regular
17. Withdraw _____ units of regular insulin from the vial and remove the needle and syringe from the regular insulin vial.	10
18. _____ the needle.	Change

19. Insert the new needle and syringe
into the NPH insulin vial and

withdraw _____ units to   25
a total of 35 units of insulin in the
syringe (a mixture of 25 units NPH
and 10 units regular).

20. *Always inject air in the longer-*
acting insulin vial first. Withdraw
the shorter-acting insulin first, then
the longer-acting insulin. If the
shorter-acting insulin is
accidentally injected into the vial
containing the longer-acting insulin,
the shorter-acting insulin will be
absorbed. The longer-acting insulin
cannot be absorbed by the shorter-
acting insulin.

Example:
The order reads 5 U regular insulin
and 30 U NPH insulin in A.M. On
hand is insulin with 100 units/cc.

Fill in the blanks.

Draw _____ units of air   30
into the insulin syringe.

21. Inject the air into the _____   NPH

insulin vial and _____   remove
the needle and syringe from the
vial.

22. Draw 5 units of air into the syringe

    and inject into the _____   regular
    insulin vial.

23. Withdraw _____ units of regular   5
    insulin.

24. Change the needle and insert the
    needle and syringe into the

    _____ insulin vial.   NPH

25. Withdraw _____ units of NPH to   30

    a total of _____ units of insulin.   35

Here are a few practice problems. Go through all the steps of mixing medications in a syringe. Determine the amount of solution to be used and the type of syringe needed. Then explain how to mix the solution in the syringe.

26. Order reads: "Meperidine 75 mg IM; hydroxyzine 25 mg IM." Meperidine comes 100 mg/ml. Hydroxyzine comes 100 mg/2 ml.

Use a 3 cc hypodermic syringe:

Draw back $\frac{3}{4}$ ml (0.75 ml or M. 12).

$$\frac{D}{H} = \frac{75 \, \cancel{mg}}{100 \, \cancel{mg}/ml} = \frac{3}{4} ml$$

Inject $\frac{3}{4}$ ml into the meperidine vial and remove the needle and syringe.

Draw back $\frac{1}{2}$ ml. $\frac{D}{H} = \frac{x}{2 \, ml}$

25 mg : 100 mg : : x : 2 ml

50 ml = 100x

$$x = \frac{1}{2} ml$$

Insert the needle and syringe in the hydroxyzine vial and inject $\frac{1}{2}$ ml air.

Withdraw $\frac{1}{2}$ ml hydroxyzine and remove the needle and syringe.

Change the needle.
Insert the new needle and syringe into the meperidine vial and remove 0.75 ml of meperidine to a total of $1\frac{1}{4}$ ml of medication in the syringe.

27. Order reads: "Regular insulin 15 U, NPH insulin 35 U SC." On hand is regular insulin 100 U/ml and NPH insulin 100 U/ml.

Use an insulin syringe.

Inject 35 units of air into the NPH insulin vial.

Remove the needle and syringe from the NPH insulin vial.

Inject 15 units of air into the regular insulin vial.

Remove 15 units of regular insulin and remove the needle and syringe from the regular insulin vial.

Change the needle.

Insert the new needle and syringe into the NPH insulin vial and remove 35 units to a total of 50 units of insulin mixed in the syringe.

28. Order reads: "Morphine sulfate 10 mg IM and atropine sulfate 0.4 mg IM." On hand is morphine sulfate 10 mg/ml and atropine sulfate 1 mg/ml.

Use a 3 cc hypodermic syringe.

Draw back 1 ml.

$$\frac{D}{H} = \frac{10 \text{ mg}}{10 \text{ mg/ml}} = 1 \text{ ml}$$

Inject 1 ml of air into the morphine sulfate vial and remove the needle and syringe.

Draw back 0.4 ml.

$$\frac{D}{H} = \frac{0.4 \text{ mg}}{1.0 \text{ mg/ml}} = 0.4 \text{ ml}$$

Insert the needle and syringe in the atropine sulfate vial.

Inject 0.4 ml of air into the atropine sulfate vial.

Withdraw 0.4 ml of atropine sulfate and remove the needle and syringe.

Change the needle.

Insert the new needle and syringe into the morphine sulfate vial and remove 10 mg (1 ml) to a total of 1.4 ml medication in the syringe.

---

29. Order reads: "Regular insulin 5 units SC, NPH insulin 42 units SC." On hand is regular insulin 100 U/ml and NPH insulin 100 U/ml.

Use an insulin syringe.

Inject 42 units of air into the NPH insulin vial.

Remove the needle and syringe from the NPH insulin vial.

Inject 5 units of air into the regular insulin vial.

Remove 5 units of regular insulin and remove the needle and syringe from the regular insulin vial.

Change the needle.

Insert the new needle and syringe into the NPH insulin vial and remove 42 units of NPH insulin to a total of 47 units.

12

Preparing Solutions

When providing care, you may need to prepare a solution or teach someone else how to do it. Solutions are commonly used for such purposes as irrigations or soaks and, depending on the situation, may be sterile or unsterile. A solution is a liquid containing a dissolved substance. It is made by dissolving one or more substances in a liquid (the solvent). These substances (solutes) may be in the form of a gas, a liquid, or a solid and may be the pure drug or the drug in a concentrated solution.

The strength of the solution is expressed as a percentage or as a ratio. Percentage indicates the amount of the drug present in 100 parts of the solution. It is a fraction, the numerator of which is expressed, and the denominator understood to be 100; for example, 25 percent is 25/100. Ratio is another way of indicating the relationship between the amount of the drug and the amount of the solution; for example, a 1:10 solution contains one part of the pure drug in ten parts of solution. Ratio and percentage really mean the same thing. For instance, a 25 percent solution also can be expressed as a 1:4 solution. It is important to remember when working problems in percentage and ratio that all measurements must be kept in the same system.

1. When caring for patients, you may be called on to prepare a <u>liquid or solution</u> for irrigations, soaks, or other treatments. A liquid, homogeneous mixture consisting of two or more components is called a

   _____.

   solution

2. In most common solutions, one of the components is a liquid in which the other component is dissolved. This liquid portion is referred to as the solvent, and the component

   which is _____ in it is known as the solute. The solute may be either solid or liquid.

   dissolved

3. The most commonly used solvent is water. In a sodium chloride solution, the solvent would be

   _____.

   water

4. The solute in a sodium chloride
    solution would be

    _____. To   sodium chloride
    make a physiologic saline solution,
    two teaspoons of table salt are
    dissolved in 1,000 ml of water.

5. For a solution that does need not to
    be sterile (e.g., mouth wash),
    ordinary tap water is the

    _____ most frequently   solvent
    used.

6. To make a sterile solution (for use
    on a wound) the most common

    solvent would be _____   sterile water

    _____.

7. Solutions are made from pure
    drugs, tablets, or stock solutions. A
    pure drug is an unadulterated
    substance in solid or liquid form.
    Expressed in percentage, a pure

    drug is _____.   100%

8. Tablets containing a known quantity of the pure drug may be used to make a solution. The

_____ is essentially a preparation of the pure drug.

tablet

---

9. A stock solution is a relatively strong solution from which a weaker solution can be made. Stock solutions are usually

_____ to make a weaker solution.

diluted

---

10. The strength of a solution can be expressed by percentage or ratio.

Percentage indicates:
(a) the number of grains of the drug in 100 grains
(b) the number of cc of the drug in 100.0 cc of the solution.

Thus, a 1% solution of peroxide contains 1.0 cc of peroxide in

_____ of solution (peroxide is a liquid).

100.0 cc

----

11. In 200.0 cc of a 1% solution of

    peroxide, there are _____   2.0 cc
    of the pure drug.

----

12. Ratio (when used with solutions)
    denotes the relative amounts of
    solute and solvent. Here the metric
    system is almost always used.

    Thus: 1:1,000 indicates 1.0 g or 1.0
    cc of pure drug in each 1,000.0 cc
    of solution.

    2:1,000 therefore indicates 2.0 g (or

    2.0 cc) of _____   pure drug

    _____ in 1,000.0 cc of
    solution.

----

13. A solution labeled 1.0 mg:1,000 ml

    contains _____ solute in   1.0 mg

    _____ solution.   1,000 ml

----

14. Now, let's work some problems in which the strength of the solution is expressed in percentage.

    The formula to be used is:

    $$\frac{\text{Desired}}{\text{On-hand}} = \frac{\text{Quantity of solute} \left(x\right)}{\text{Quantity of solution} \left(V\right)}$$

    or

    $$\frac{D}{H} = \frac{x}{V}$$

    Example
    How many cc of pure drug will be needed to prepare 1 liter of a 40% solution? How will you prepare the solution?

    $$\frac{D}{H} = \frac{x}{V}$$

    Substitute known values:

    $$\frac{40\%}{\underline{\quad ? \quad}} = \frac{x}{1,000.0 \text{ cc}} \left(1.0 \text{ liter}\right)$$

    100%

15. $$\frac{40\%}{100\%} = \frac{x}{\underline{\quad ? \quad}}$$

    1,000.0 cc

16. $100x = 40,000.0$ cc

    $x = $ _____

    400.0 cc of pure drug will be needed

---

17. To prepare the 40% solution of
    drug, place the 400.0 cc of pure
    drug in a container and add water

    to make _____.   1,000.0 cc

---

18. Example:

    Prepare 250.0 cc of a 1% neomycin
    sulfate solution. How much
    neomycin sulfate will be needed?
    How will you prepare the solution?
    Use the formula:

    $$\frac{D}{H} = \frac{x}{V}$$

    $$\frac{1\%}{100\%} = \frac{?}{?}$$ $$\frac{x}{250.0 \text{ cc}}$$

---

19. $$\frac{1\%}{100\%} = \frac{x}{250.0 \text{ cc}}$$

    Finish calculations and label
    answer.
                                        $100x = 250.0$ cc
                                        $x = 2.5$ cc of neomycin
                                        sulfate will be needed. To
                                        this amount of drug add
                                        water to make 250.0 cc of
                                        solution. This is a 1%
                                        solution.

---

20. One more example:
5.0 g of boric acid for a sterile solution is dispensed. How much 5% solution can be made from one vial?

Note: In this problem, the amount of solute is known rather than the amount of solution to be made.

The same basic formula is used:

$$\frac{D}{H} = \frac{V}{x}\frac{(\text{quantity of solute})}{(\text{quantity of solution})}$$

$$\frac{5\%}{100\%} = \frac{5.0 \text{ g or cc}}{x}$$

Finish calculations and label answer.

$$5x = 500.0 \text{ cc}$$
$$x = 100.0 \text{ cc}$$
It is stated in the volume unit rather than solid unit. The 5.0 g of boric acid is dissolved in 100.0 cc of sterile water—100.0 cc of a 5% boric acid solution.

---

21. From a 3% hydrogen peroxide
    solution, how will you prepare 1
    ounce of a 1% solution?

$$\frac{D}{H} = \frac{x}{V}$$

$$\frac{1\%}{3\%} = \frac{x}{30.0 \text{ cc}^*}$$

*(equivalent of
1 fluid ounce)

$3x = 30.0$ cc

$x = 10.0$ cc of 3% hydrogen
peroxide solution is needed.
Add water to make 30.0 cc
(1 fluid ounce). You now
have 1 ounce of 1%
hydrogen peroxide
solution.

---

22. How will you make 1 quart of a
    10% solution of neomycin sulfate?

$$\frac{D}{H} = \frac{x}{V}$$

$$\frac{10\%}{100\%} = \frac{x}{1,000.0 \text{ cc}^*}$$

*(equivalent of 1 quart)

$100x = 10,000.0$ cc

$x = 100.0$ cc neomycin
sulfate is needed. Add
water to make 1,000 cc
(1 quart). You now have
1 quart of 10% neomycin
sulfate solution.

---

23. How much hydrochloric acid will be needed to make 2 liters of a 2% solution?

$$\frac{D}{H} = \frac{x}{V}$$

$$\frac{2\%}{100\%} = \frac{x}{2,000.0 \text{ cc}}$$

$100x = 4,000.0$ cc

$x = 40.0$ cc of hydrochloric acid is needed. Add water to make 2,000.0 cc. You now have 2 liters of 2% hydrochloric acid solution.

24. How will you make 200.0 ml of a 1:40 acetic acid solution from a 1:20 acetic acid solution?

$$\frac{D}{H} = \frac{x}{V}$$

$$\frac{1/40}{1/20} = \frac{x}{200.0 \text{ ml}}$$

$$\frac{1}{20}x = 200.0 \text{ ml} \times \frac{1}{40}$$

$x = 100.0$ ml of 1:20 acetic acid solution is needed. Add water to make 200.0 ml of 1:40 acetic acid solution.

---

25. When the strength of the solution is expressed in ratio, this formula will be used:

$$\frac{\text{Desired ratio}}{\text{On-hand ratio}} = \frac{\text{Quantity of solute}}{\text{Quantity of solution}}$$

or

$$\frac{D}{H} = \frac{?}{\underline{\quad ? \quad}}$$

$$\frac{x}{V}$$

---

26. Example:
How much solute is needed to make 2,000.0 ml of a 1:5,000 sodium bicarbonate solution from a 1:1,000 solution?

$$\frac{D}{H} = \frac{x}{V}$$

$$\frac{1:5,000}{1:1,000} = \frac{?}{\underline{\quad ? \quad}}$$

$$\frac{x}{2,000.0 \text{ ml}}$$

---

27. $\dfrac{1/5,000}{1/1,000} = \dfrac{x}{2,000.0 \text{ ml}}$

$\dfrac{1}{1,000\,x} = 2,000.0 \text{ ml} \times \dfrac{1}{5,000}$

$x = \underline{\hspace{2cm}}.$

Finish calculations and label answer.

$x = \dfrac{2}{5}\text{ml} \div \dfrac{1}{1,000}$

$x = 400.0 \text{ ml of the } \dfrac{1}{1,000}$

sodium bicarbonate solution will be needed (Note: Here, the problem asks only how much drug will be needed)

---

28. Example:
How will you prepare 1 quart of 1:20 solution of boric acid from the crystals?

$\dfrac{D}{H} = \dfrac{x}{V}$

$\dfrac{1/20}{1/1} = \dfrac{x}{1,000.0 \text{ cc}}$

(This is the equivalent of one quart)

$1x = 1,000.0 \text{ cc} \times \dfrac{1}{20}$

$x = \underline{\hspace{1.5cm}}$ of boric acid crystals will be needed. Add water to make

$\underline{\hspace{4cm}}$ solution.
You now have one quart of 1:20 solution of boric acid.

50 g

1,000.0 cc (1 quart)
(Note: This problem asks how you will prepare the solution.)

29. How much stock solution of benzalkonium chloride 1:1,000 is needed to make 1 liter of 1:10,000 solution?

$$\frac{D}{H} = \frac{x}{V}$$

$$\frac{1/10,000}{1/1,000} = \frac{x}{1,000.0 \text{ cc}}$$

$$\frac{1}{1,000.0} x = 1,000.0 \text{ cc} \times \frac{1}{10,000}$$

x = 100.0 cc of 1:1,000 benzalkonium chloride solution is needed

30. Make 1 gallon of 5% boric acid solution from a 1:5 boric acid solution.

1 gallon = 4,000.0 cc
Change 5% to its ratio equivalent 1:20

$(5\% = \dfrac{5}{100} = \dfrac{1}{20}$ = 1:20. Do you need to review this process?)

$$\frac{D}{H} = \frac{x}{V}$$

$$\frac{1/20}{1/5} = \frac{x}{4,000.0 \text{ cc}}$$

$$\frac{1}{5} x = 4,000.0 \text{ cc} \times \frac{1}{20}$$

x = 1,000.0 cc of 1:5 boric acid solution is needed to make 4,000.0 cc (1 gallon). You now have 1 gallon of 5% boric acid solution.

13

Administering Intravenous Medications

Fluids and electrolyte solutions are often administered by intravenous infusion. The safe and therapeutic administration of any solution is very important.

The purpose of this chapter is to help you develop the skills necessary to calculate proper flow rates and to determine the amount of fluid or drug the patient is receiving in a specific period of time. It will also acquaint you with your responsibility when medication is being given via a pump.

1. When an order for <u>fluid administration</u> is written it should include the solution to be administered and the rate of administration. Usually the order will be written thus:

    "1,000 cc D$_5$W q 8 hours IV" indicating that 1,000 cc of D$_5$W is to

    be infused over a period of _____ hours.

    8

2. To further simplify, determine the amount of fluid to be administered in one hour using the following formula:

    Total amount ÷ total time = amount to be administered in one hour.

    In the above example: 1,000 cc ÷ 8 =

    _____ cc administered in 1 hour.

    125

3. Parenteral administration sets deliver fluids by drops (via a drip chamber) that vary in size.

    The larger the size of the drop, the fewer the number of drops that will be needed to administer 1 cc. The smaller the size of the drop, the

    _____ the number of drops that will be needed to administer 1 cc.

    greater

4. Information on drop size is available from the manufacturer of the equipment, and should be indicated on the set. This is called the drop factor. Example: A set labeled with a drop factor of 10 will

   need _____ drops to administer 1 cc of the solution.

   10

---

5. A drop factor of 15 indicates the set will deliver 1 cc of fluid for every

   _____ drops.

   15

---

6. When the drop factor is known, the drops per minute necessary to administer a specific amount of fluid in a prescribed time period is easily calculated by using the following formula:

   $$\text{Drops / min} = \frac{\text{Total cc} \times \text{drop factor}}{\text{minutes}}$$

   In the previous example, the number of cc to be administered IV in 1 hour was determined:

   1,000 cc ÷ 8 = _____

   125 cc per hour

7. Next, using a drop factor of 10, set
   up the formula:

   $$\text{Drops / min} = \frac{\text{Total cc} \times \text{drop factor}}{\text{minutes}}$$

   $$x = \frac{125 \text{ cc} \times \underline{\quad ? \quad}}{60 \text{ minutes}}$$

   10

8. Solve for x.

   $$x = \frac{125 \times 10}{60}$$

   $$x = \frac{125}{6}$$

   $x = 20.8$ or
   $= 21$ drops/min to deliver
   125 cc in 1 hour or
   1,000 cc in 8 hours

9. Try another problem. The order
   reads "Administer by IV 500 cc
   D_5W in 8 hours." A check of your
   equipment indicates the drop factor
   to be 10. Now you have all the
   information necessary to determine

   the flow rate, or the _____

   number of drops
   per minute

   _____ _____

   _____ _____.

10. Take it step by step. First, determine the amount of solution to be delivered in one hour:

Total amount ÷ total time = amount per minute.

or

500 cc ÷ 8 hours = _____.

62.5 cc

---

11. The drop factor given above is

_____.

10

---

12. The time (in minutes) is _____.

60

---

13. Using the flow rate formula

Drops/min =

$$\frac{\text{Amount in cc} \times \text{drop factor}}{\text{time in minutes}}$$

Substitute known values and solve for x.

$$x = \frac{62.5 \text{ cc} \times 10}{60 \text{ min}}$$

$x = 62.5 \div 6$

$x = 10.4$ or 10 drops/min to administer 62.5 cc fluid in 1 hour or 500 cc in 8 hours

14. Order: "200 cc 0.9 NaCl IV in 2 hours." The drop factor is 15. What is the flow rate per minute?

$$200 \text{ cc} \div 2 \text{ hours}$$
$$= 100 \text{ cc in 1 hour}$$
$$x = \frac{100 \times 15}{60}$$
$$x = 100 \div 4$$

$x = 25$ drops/min to administer 100 cc 0.9 NaCl in 1 hour or 200 cc in 2 hours

15. It is frequently necessary to administer very small quantities of fluid over a period of time (for example, to infants or when very potent drugs are being given). To facilitate this, the flow is measured in microdrops per minute. Most of the sets used for this purpose have drop chambers that deliver 60 microdrops per cc. These sets are designated as Pedi-sets or Microdrip sets.

The flow rate for a Microdrip set is

_____.

60

16. Use the flow rate formula to implement the following order: "100 cc of 10% glucose in D_5W by intravenous to a 10-month-old over 4 hours."

100 cc in 4 hours = _____ in 1 hour.

25 cc

17. Using a Pedi-set, delivering 60 drops per cc, substitute known values in the formula and solve for x.

$$Microdrops/min = \frac{Total\ amount \times drop\ factor}{Time}$$

$$x = \frac{25\ cc \times 60}{60\ minutes}$$

$x = 25$ microdrops/min to deliver 25 cc in 1 hour or 100 cc in 4 hours.

18. Here is another order:
"Give 500 cc 0.45 NaCl by IV in 10 hours." The Microdrop set has a drop factor of 60.

You will regulate the set to run at what microdrops/min?

$$500 \text{ cc} \div 10$$
$$= 50 \text{ cc in one hour}$$
$$x = \frac{50 \text{ cc} \times 60}{60 \text{ minutes}}$$

x = 50 microdrops/min to administer 50 cc in 1 hour or 500 cc in 10 hours

Easy, isn't it? If you did make an error, please go back to frame 6 and identify the error.

---

19. You may have noted in the above examples that when using a Pedi-set or Micro-set delivering 60 drops/cc, the number of cc delivered each hour is equal to the number of drops per minute.

Therefore, when using a set that delivers 60 drops per cc you will not need to calculate the flow rate by the previous formula. Instead, consider:

Drops/min = cc/hour

or

15 drops/min = _____ cc/hour

REMEMBER: Before using this short-cut, be sure the set you are using delivers 60 drops/cc.

15

20. Give 800 cc lactated Ringer's solution IV in 4 hours using a drop factor of 10. What is the flow rate to be used?

$$800 \text{ cc} \div 4 \text{ hours} = 200 \text{ cc in 1 hour}$$

$$\text{Flow rate} = \frac{\text{Total cc} \times \text{drop factor}}{\text{Time in minutes}}$$

$$x = \frac{200 \text{ cc} \times 10}{60}$$

$$x = 200 \div 6$$

$$x = 33\frac{1}{3} \text{ or } 33 \text{ drops/min to}$$

administer 200 cc lactated Ringer's solution IV in 1 hour or 800 cc in 4 hours

21. Your postoperative hysterectomy client has an order for 2,500 cc D_5 in $\frac{1}{2}$ NSS to be given IV every 12 hours. Your IV set has a drop factor of 15. You will adjust the set to deliver

_____ drops per minute.

$$2,500 \text{ cc} \div 12 \text{ hours} = 208 \text{ cc per 1 hour}$$

$$\text{Flow rate} = \frac{\text{Total cc} \times \text{drop factor}}{\text{Time in minutes}}$$

$$x = \frac{208 \times 15}{60}$$

$$x = 208 \div 4$$

$$x = 52 \text{ drops/min to administer}$$

208 cc D_5 in $\frac{1}{2}$ NSS IV in 1 hour or 2,500 cc in 12 hours

22. Give 1,000 cc NSS by IV in 10 hours. The drop factor is 15. What is the flow rate?

$$1,000 \text{ cc} \div 10 \text{ hours} =$$
$$100 \text{ cc in 1 hour}$$
$$x = \frac{100 \times 15}{60}$$
$$x = 100 \div 4$$
$$x = 25 \text{ drops/min to}$$
administer 100 cc NSS by IV in 1 hour or 1,000 cc in 10 hours

23. Give an infant 120 cc physiologic saline IV in 6 hours. The drop factor is 60. What is the flow rate?

$$120 \text{ cc} \div 6 \text{ hours} =$$
$$20 \text{ cc in 1 hour}$$
$$x = \frac{20 \times 60}{60}$$
$$x = 20 \text{ drops/min to}$$
administer 20 cc physiologic saline in 1 hour or 120 cc in 6 hours

24. Your postcholecystectomy client is to receive 250 cc packed cells in 2 hours. The blood administration set states "6 drops per cc." The flow rate will be:

$$250 \text{ cc} \div 2 \text{ hours} = 125 \text{ cc}$$
$$\text{in 1 hour}$$
$$x = \frac{125 \times 6}{60}$$
$$x = 12.5 \text{ or } 13 \text{ drops/min}$$
to administer 125 cc packed cells in 1 hour or 250 cc in 2 hours

25. Sometimes an IV medication is ordered to be infused by a dose and you must calculate the flow rate. (To calculate the flow rate, a proportion must be used.)

    For example, an order reads: "Heparin 2,000 units/hr from an IV solution of 20,000 units of heparin in 1,000 cc NSS."

    How many ml/hr are to be infused?

    $$\frac{20{,}000 \text{ units}}{\underline{\quad ? \quad} \text{ cc}} = \frac{2{,}000 \text{ units/hr}}{x \text{ cc}}$$

    1,000

---

26. $1{,}000 \times 2{,}000 = \underline{\hspace{3cm}} x$

    20,000

    $2{,}000{,}000 = 20{,}000x$

    $2{,}000{,}000 \times 20{,}000 = x \text{ cc/hr}$

    $x = \underline{\hspace{2cm}} \text{ cc/hr}$

    100

---

27. Another example is: Pitocin is ordered to run at 0.02 units per minute from an IV solution of 10 units/1,000 ml PSS. How many ml/hr are to be infused?

    The first thing that must be done is to convert units/min to units/hr.

    $0.02 \text{ U/min} = \underline{\hspace{3cm}} \text{ U/hr}$

    $0.02 \times 60 = 1.2$

28. $\dfrac{10 \text{ U}}{1,000 \text{ cc}} = \dfrac{1.2 \text{ U}}{x \text{ cc}}$

$1,200 = 10x$

$1,200 \div \underline{\hspace{1.5cm}} = x \text{ cc/hr}$ 10

$x = \underline{\hspace{1.5cm}} \text{ cc/hr}$ 120

29. It may also be necessary to calculate hourly doses of medication when the hourly volume to be infused has been ordered. IT IS YOUR RESPONSIBILITY TO KNOW THE DOSAGE OF THE MEDICATION BEING ADMINISTERED.

For example, an order reads: "IV 1,000 cc PSS with 20,000 units of heparin to infuse at 100 cc/hr."

To calculate the dose that the patient receives every hour, a proportion is used.

$\dfrac{20,000 \text{ U}}{1,000 \text{ cc}} = \dfrac{x \text{ U}}{100 \text{ cc}}$

$x = \underline{\hspace{3cm}}$ 2,000 U/hr

30. Heparin 2,500 units an hour from an IV solution of 20,000 units in 1,000 cc NSS. How many cc per hour are to be infused?

$$\frac{20{,}000 \text{ U}}{1{,}000 \text{ cc}} = \frac{2{,}500 \text{ U}}{x \text{ cc}}$$

$$2{,}500{,}000 = 20{,}000x$$
$$250 \div 2 = x \text{ cc/hr}$$
$$x = 125 \text{ cc/hr}$$

31. The order reads: 500 mg of aminophylline in 250 cc D$_5$/W to run at 10 cc/hr. What is the dose that the patient receives in 1 hour?

$$\frac{500 \text{ mg}}{250 \text{ cc}} = \frac{x \text{ mg}}{10 \text{ cc}}$$

$$5{,}000 = 250x$$
$$5{,}000 \div 250 = x$$
$$x = 20 \text{ mg aminophylline}$$
$$\text{in 1 hour}$$

32. IV pumps and IV controllers are also available. These are used for IV medications that must be delivered at an exact rate at all times. These pumps or controllers would be used

   if a _____ *must* be given at a set rate. Examples are lidocaine, aminophylline, and heparin.

   medication

   Each manufacturer includes specific instructions with the machines. It is essential to acquaint yourself with the machine and the set-up before using it.

   Some IV medications are given through sets that control the volume. These volume-control sets are called Buretrol, Soluset, Volutrol, Peditrol. The manufacturer provides detailed instructions (usually included in the package). Read the directions carefully before using.

33. Intravenous medications may be ordered to run with another medication. This is called piggyback.

If an IV medication is run with another IV it is called

_____.

piggyback

---

34. The medication that is piggybacked is usually dissolved in another 50 to 100 cc of a solution.

The medication is dissolved in

50 to 100 cc of _____.

solution

---

35. The instructions usually tell you how long the medication should run.

For example, the order reads: Amoxicillin 500 mg in 50 cc D5W to run for 30 minutes.

The _____ cc would be infused

50

in _____ minutes.

30

36. The calculation of the drops
     per minute would be done as
     previously explained. The
     formula is:

$$\text{drops/min} = \frac{\text{total cc} \times \text{drop factor}}{\text{minutes}}$$

37. This set delivers 15 drops per
     cc. Calculate the drops per
     minute for the example in
     frame 35.

$$\text{drops/min} = \frac{50 \text{ cc} \times 15 \text{ gtts/cc}}{30 \text{ minutes}}$$

$$= \frac{75 \text{ gtts}}{30 \text{ min}}$$

$$= 25 \text{ gtts/min}$$

Medications for Infants and Children

Medications can be administered to infants and children by any of the routes used for adults. When administering medications to infants and children, the dosage must be carefully calculated based on body weight in kilograms. While the dose of the medication will be specified on the prescription, it is important for the individual administering the medication to be certain that the correct dose has been prescribed. This requires calculating the body weight in kilograms and then calculating the correct dosage.

The pediatric dose is listed in various drug references and in package inserts. In addition to the listing of the dose per kilogram, an upper limit of the drug that can be administered to the child is stated.

In this chapter, you will learn how to calculate the amount of medication to be given to an infant or child. A child over 12 years of age is usually considered an adult and is given the adult dose.

1. While the dose of the drug will be ordered by the provider, it is important for the person administering the drug to recognize whether the dose is within safe _____.

limits (or range)

2. In drug references, the correct pediatric dosage of the drug that can be administered is given along with the _____ _____ of the drug that can be safely administered.

upper limit

3. The correct dosage of the drug is calculated based on the _____ _____ of the child.

body weight

4. The body weight of the child is calculated in _____.

kilograms

5. Ibuprofen (Motrin) suspension every 6 hours is ordered for a child who weighs 36 pounds. The bottle reads 100 mg/5 ml. The insert reads that the correct dose is 10 mg/kg every 6 hours to a maxium of 40/mg/kg/day.

    To determine the correct dose, the body weight of the child is calculated in kilograms. The body

    weight in kilograms is _____ _____ kilograms.

    $36 \div 2.2 = 16.3636 = 16.37$

6. The next step is to calculate the correct dosage.

    dosage = weight (in kg) × mg/kg =

    _____ kg × _____ mg/kg

    16.37 kg × 10 mg/kg

7. Correct dose = 16.37 kg × 10 mg/kg =

    _____ mg

    163.7

8. The child would receive 164 mg. The medication comes 100 mg/5 ml so the correct volume must be calculated. To do this the formula, $\frac{D}{H} \times V$ is used.

The D (desired) dose is _____ mg.

164

9. The H (on-hand) medication is

_____ mg/5 ml.

100

10. The dose per ml is then calculated. This is done by dividing the dose by the number of ml. The formula is:

$$\frac{D}{H} \times V$$

11. The correct dose is:

$$\frac{164 \text{ mg}}{100 \text{ mg}} \times 5 \text{ ml} = 8.2 \text{ ml}$$

---

12.   This means that the child should

receive _____ ml of   8.2
Motrin 100 mg/5 ml every 6 hours.

---

13.   Another way that pediatric
medication dosage may be
presented is the amount per
kilogram for 24 hours.

A 22 pound infant is prescribed
amoxicillin suspension t.i.d. The
package insert reads 20 mg/kg/day
in 3 divided doses. The medicine is
dispensed as 125 mg/5 ml.

The first step in calculating the
correct dose is to determine the

body weight in _____.   kilograms

---

14.   The correct formula to calculate the
body weight in kilograms is:

$$\frac{\text{pounds}}{\text{kilograms/pound}}$$

22
2.2

---

15.   The child's weight is _____   10
kilograms.

---

16. The next step is to calculate the correct dose per day. The recommended dose is 20 mg/kg/day. Since the child weighs 10 kilograms, he

    should receive _____

    _____ mg in 24 hours.

    20 mg/kg × 10 kg = 200 mg

17. Since 200 mg is to be given over an entire day and the child is to receive 3 doses a day, the correct amount for each dose must be calculated. This is done by using

    the equation _____.

    $$\frac{200 \text{ mg}}{3}$$

18. The correct dose at each

    administration is _____ mg.

    66.67 = 67

19. Since the medication comes in 125 mg/5 ml, the correct volume must be calculated. The formula

    _____ is used.

    $$\frac{D}{H} \times V$$

20. When substituting the numbers, the formula is

_____.

$$\frac{67\ mg}{125\ mg} \times 5\ ml$$

---

21. The correct volume of medication is _____ ml for each administration.

$$2.68 = 2.7$$

---

22. Tylenol (acetaminophen) is ordered every 6 hours for a child weighing 36 pounds. The bottle reads 240 mg every 4–6 hours for a child 30–40 lbs. The strength of the medicine is 160 mg/5 ml. How much would you give?

$$\frac{D}{H} \times V = \frac{240\ mg}{160\ mg} \times 5\ ml = 7.5\ ml$$

---

23. Zithromax (azythromycin) is ordered for a child weighing 30 pounds. The recommended dose is 12 mg/kg/day. The medication comes 200 mg/5 ml. How much would you give daily?

$$30\ pounds = 13.64\ kg$$
$$13.64\ kg \times 12\ mg/kg/day = 163.68\ mg/day$$

$$\frac{D}{H} \times V = \frac{163.68\ mg}{200\ mg} \times 5\ ml = 4.0$$
(rounded off)

24. Slo-phyllin (theophylline) is ordered for a 6-month-old weighing 19 pounds. The recommended dose is 4 mg/kg/dose. It comes 80 mg/15 ml. What dose would you give?

$$19 \text{ pounds} = 8.64 \text{ kg}$$
$$8.64 \text{ kg} \times 4 \text{ mg/kg} = 34.5 \text{ mg}$$
$$\frac{D}{H} \times V = \frac{34.5 \text{ mg}}{80 \text{ mg}} \times 15 \text{ ml} = 6.5 \text{ ml}$$

25. Ceclor (cefaclor) is ordered for a 40-pound child. The recommended dose is 40 mg/kg/day in 3 divided doses. It comes 250 mg/5 ml. How much would you give at each dose?

$$40 \text{ pounds} = 18.18 \text{ kg}$$
$$18.18 \text{ kg} \times 40 \text{ mg/kg/day} = 727.2 \text{ mg/day}$$

$$\frac{727.2 \text{ mg/day}}{3} = 242.4 \text{ mg/dose}$$

$$\frac{D}{H} \times V = \frac{242.4 \text{ mg}}{250 \text{ mg}} \times 5 \text{ ml}$$

$$= .97 \times 5 \text{ ml} = 4.85 \text{ ml} = 5 \text{ ml}$$
(rounded off)

Post Test

Comprehensive Self-Examination

Directions: Place the correct letter in the space provided.

1. 60.0 kg = _____ g

   a. 0.006 g
   b. 0.06 g
   c. 600.0 g
   d. 6,000.0 g
   e. 60,000.0 g

1. e

2. 75.0 mg = _____ g

   a. 7,500.0 g
   b. 750.0 g
   c. 0.75 g
   d. 0.075 g
   e. 0.0075 g

2. d

3. 25.0 ml = _____ cc

   a. 2.5 cc
   b. 25.0 cc
   c. 250.0 cc
   d. 500.0 cc
   e. 2,500.0 cc

3. b

4. 55.0 liters = _____ ml

   a. 0.055 ml
   b. 0.05 ml
   c. 0.5 ml
   d. 5,500.0 ml
   e. 55,000.0 ml

4. e

5.   25.4 cm = _____ inch(es)

    a.   1 inch
    b.   5 inches
    c.   10 inches
    d.   12 inches
    e.   15 inches

5.   c

6.   12 inches = _____ cm

    a.   25 cm
    b.   28 cm
    c.   30.5 cm
    d.   31.2 cm
    e.   36 cm

6.   c

7. $32°C =$ _____ $°F$

    a. $86.2°F$
    b. $87.6°F$
    c. $89.6°F$
    d. $95°F$
    e. $98.6°F$

7.   c

8. $100°F =$ _____ $°C$

    a. $34°C$
    b. $36.2°C$
    c. $37°C$
    d. $37.8°C$
    e. $39°C$

8.   d

9. ounces 48 = pints _____

    a. 2 pints
    b. 3 pints
    c. 4 pints
    d. 6 pints
    e. 7 pints

9. b

---

10. quarts 10 = pints _____

    a. 5 pints
    b. 15 pints
    c. 20 pints
    d. 25 pints
    e. 30 pints

10. c

---

11. 240 drops = _____ teaspoonful(s)

    a. 1 teaspoonful
    b. 2 teaspoonfuls
    c. 3 teaspoonfuls
    d. 4 teaspoonfuls
    e. 5 teaspoonfuls

11. d

---

12. 5 tablespoonfuls = _____ teaspoonfuls

    a. 10 teaspoonfuls
    b. 15 teaspoonfuls
    c. 20 teaspoonfuls
    d. 25 teaspoonfuls
    e. 30 teaspoonfuls

12. b

---

13.   3 ounces = _____ tablespoonfuls

    a.   2 tablespoonfuls
    b.   4 tablespoonfuls
    c.   6 tablespoonfuls
    d.   8 tablespoonfuls
    e.   10 tablespoonfuls

13. c

---

14.   5.0 g = gr _____

    a.   gr 15
    b.   gr 30
    c.   gr 45
    d.   gr 60
    e.   gr 75

14. e

---

15.   180.0 g = ounces (oz) _____

    a.   6 oz
    b.   10 oz
    c.   250 oz
    d.   540 oz
    e.   5,400 oz

15. a

---

16.   ℨxxx = _____ cc

    a.   90 cc
    b.   260 cc
    c.   500 cc
    d.   750 cc
    e.   900 cc

16. e

---

17. 4.2 cc = M _____   **17.** e

    a. 23 M
    b. 40 M
    c. 48 M
    d. 60 M
    e. 63 M

18. 150 pounds = _____ kg   **18.** d

    a. 90 kg
    b. 149.6 kg
    c. 76 kg
    d. 68 kg
    e. 40 kg

19. 21 kg = _____ pounds   **19.** d

    a. 40 pounds
    b. 42 pounds
    c. 45.8 pounds
    d. 46.2 pounds
    e. 47 pounds

20. You are to administer Gantrisin 1.0 g. The tablets you have are labeled Gantrisin 0.5 g. How many tablet(s) will you administer?

    _____

    a. $\frac{1}{2}$ tablet
    b. 1 tablet
    c. $1\frac{1}{2}$ tablets
    d. 2 tablets
    e. $2\frac{1}{2}$ tablets

20. d

21. You are to administer phenobarbital 90.0 mg. The tablets you have are labeled phenobarbital gr ss. How many tablet(s) will you administer? _____

    a. 1 tablet
    b. 2 tablets
    c. 3 tablets
    d. 4 tablets
    e. 5 tablets

21. c

22. You have an oral medication bottle labeled "Elixir of Donnatol ℨi = gr xv." Your doctor ordered you to take gr xxx. How many

teaspoonful(s) will you take? _____   **22.** c

   a. $\frac{1}{2}$ teaspoonful
   b. 1 teaspoonful
   c. 2 teaspoonfuls
   d. 3 teaspoonfuls
   e. $3\frac{1}{2}$ teaspoonfuls

23. You are to give sulfasuxidine 2.0 g. The tablets you have are labeled sulfasuxidine 500 mg.

How many tablet(s) will you give? _____   **23.** e

   a. 0.25 tablet
   b. 1.0 tablet
   c. 2.25 tablets
   d. 3.0 tablets
   e. 4.0 tablets

24. You are to give A.S.A. 300 mg. The tablets you have are labeled A.S.A. 0.3 g. How many

tablet(s) will you give? _____   **24.** b

   a. $\frac{1}{2}$ tablet
   b. 1 tablet
   c. $1\frac{1}{2}$ tablets
   d. 2 tablets
   e. 5 tablets

25. You are to give Milk of Magnesia ʒi. How
    many cc is this? _____

    25. e

    a. 10 cc
    b. 15 cc
    c. 20 cc
    d. 25 cc
    e. 30 cc

26. You are to drink 1,000 cc of water in 8 hours.
    How many quarts (qt) would this be? _____

    26. b

    a. $\frac{1}{2}$ qt
    b. 1 qt
    c. $1\frac{1}{2}$ qt
    d. 2 qt
    e. $2\frac{1}{2}$ qt

27. You are to give digitalis leaf 90 mg. The
    tablets you have are labeled 60 mg. How many
    tablet(s) will you give? _____

    27. c

    a. $\frac{1}{2}$ tablet
    b. 1 tablet
    c. $1\frac{1}{2}$ tablets
    d. 2 tablets
    e. $2\frac{1}{2}$ tablets

28. You are to administer penicillin 750,000 units intramuscularly. The bottle of penicillin is labeled 300,000 units/cc. How many cc will

you administer? _____   **28.** d

   a. 0.4 cc
   b. 0.8 cc
   c. 1.5 cc
   d. 2.5 cc
   e. 3.5 cc

29. You have Ancef containing 500.0 mg in 1.0 cc. You are to give 400.0 mg. How much solution

will you give? _____   **29.** c

   a. 0.2 cc
   b. 0.5 cc
   c. 0.8 cc
   d. 1.25 cc
   e. 1.55 cc

30. You have a solution of cortisone acetate 25.0 mg in 1.0 cc. You are to give 60.0 mg.

How much solution will you give? _____   **30.** d

   a. 0.4 cc
   b. 0.8 cc
   c. 1.8 cc
   d. 2.4 cc
   e. 3.2 cc

31. You are to give 50 units of regular insulin.
     You have on hand a bottle labeled: "Regular
     insulin U-100" and a 3-ml hypodermic
     syringe. How much solution would you give?

     _____   **31.** b

     a. 0.2 cc
     b. 0.5 cc
     c. 1.2 cc
     d. 1.5 cc
     e. 2.0 cc

32. You are to give cephalothin sodium gr viiss.
     You have a vial labeled: "Cephalothin sodium
     0.5 g in 2.0 cc." How much of this solution

     would you give? _____   **32.** e

     a. 0.2 cc
     b. 0.5 cc
     c. 1.2 cc
     d. 1.5 cc
     e. 2.0 cc

33. What type of syringe would you use for the

     injection described in problem 32? _____   **33.** b

     a. tuberculin
     b. 3-ml hypodermic
     c. 5-ml hypodermic
     d. 10-ml hypodermic
     e. 30-ml hypodermic

34. You are to give 100,000 units of sodium penicillin G from a multi-dose vial labeled: "Sodium penicillin G, 1,000,000 units per 10.0 cc." How many cc will you need to use?

_____   **34.** a

  a. 1.0 cc
  b. 2.0 cc
  c. 5.0 cc
  d. 7.0 cc
  e. 10.0 cc

35. What type of syringe would you use for the

injection described in problem 34? _____   **35.** c

  a. tuberculin
  b. insulin
  c. 3-ml hypodermic
  d. 5-ml hypodermic
  e. 10-ml hypodermic

36. You are to give chlorpromazine 0.075 g from a bottle labeled: "Chlorpromazine 25.0 mg per ml." How much solution will you use?

_____   **36.** c

  a. 1.5 ml
  b. 2.0 ml
  c. 3.0 ml
  d. 3.5 ml
  e. 4.0 ml

37. You are to give atropine sulfate 0.2 mg

   (gr $\frac{1}{300}$). You have a bottle of solution
   labeled: "Atropine sulfate 0.4 mg per cc."

   How much solution will you use? _____   **37. a**

   a. 0.5 cc
   b. 1.0 cc
   c. 1.5 cc
   d. 2.0 cc
   e. 2.5 cc

38. You are to give 600,000 units of penicillin.
   You have a bottle labeled: "Penicillin
   3,000,000 units per 10.0 cc." How much

   solution will you use? _____   **38. d**

   a. 0.5 cc
   b. 1.2 cc
   c. 1.5 cc
   d. 2.0 cc
   e. 2.5 cc

39. You have a vial containing 500 units of a drug
   in dry form. How much diluent will you use
   to prepare a solution containing 125 units of
                                                 39. d
   drug per cc? _____

   a. 0.25 cc
   b. 1.0 cc
   c. 2.5 cc
   d. 4.0 cc
   e. 10.0 cc

40. A vial of potassium penicillin G contains 3,000,000 units of the dry drug. How much diluent will be needed to make a solution that contains 400,000 units of this drug per cc?

_____   **40.** e

   a. 0.25 cc
   b. 2.5 cc
   c. 5.0 cc
   d. 6.5 cc
   e. 7.5 cc

41. You have a vial containing 25.0 mg of a drug in dry form. How much diluent will you use to prepare a solution containing 2.0 mg of

drug per cc? _____   **41.** d

   a. 5.0 cc
   b. 7.5 cc
   c. 10.0 cc
   d. 12.5 cc
   e. 15.0 cc

42. You are at home and need to prepare 8 oz. of a normal saline solution (0.9% strength). How many teaspoonful(s) of table salt will you add

to 8 oz. of hot water? _____   **42.** a

   a. $\frac{1}{2}$ teaspoonful
   b. 1 teaspoonful
   c. 2 teaspoonful
   d. $2\frac{1}{2}$ teaspoonfuls
   e. 3 teaspoonfuls

43. You are to prepare 1,000.0 cc of 1:5,000
solution of potassium permanganate. You
have a stock solution labeled potassium
permanganate 1:1,000. How many cc of this

stock solution do you need? _____   **43. b**

    a.   100.0 cc
    b.   200.0 cc
    c.   300.0 cc
    d.   400.0 cc
    e.   500.0 cc

44. How many cc of diluent do you need to add
to the stock solution in problem 43 in order to
prepare the 1,000.0 cc of 1:5,000 potassium

permanganate solution? _____   **44. b**

    a.   900.0 cc
    b.   800.0 cc
    c.   700.0 cc
    d.   600.0 cc
    e.   500.0 cc

45. Give 500 cc packed cells over a period of
4 hours. Your blood set delivers 10 drops/cc.

What is the flow rate? _____   **45. c**

    a.   10 drops/min
    b.   15 drops/min
    c.   20 drops/min
    d.   25 drops/min
    e.   40 drops/min

46. Order: "100 cc lactated Ringer's solution in 8 hours." Using a Pedi-set, the flow rate will

be _____ microdrops/min.   **46.** c

    a. 8 microdrops/min
    b. 10 microdrops/min
    c. 12 microdrops/min
    d. 14 microdrops/min
    e. 30 microdrops/min

47. Order: "1,000 cc D_5W to run at a rate of 125 cc per hour." What is the flow rate if the set

delivers 15 gtt/cc? _____   **47.** c

    a. 3.1 gtt/min
    b. 6.5 gtt/min
    c. 31 gtt/min
    d. 38 gtt/min
    e. 45 gtt/min

48. Order "3,000 cc D_5W over 24 hours." What is the flow rate if the drop factor is 10 gtt/cc?

    _____   **48.** c

    a. 15 gtt/min
    b. 17 gtt/min
    c. 21 gtt/min
    d. 25 gtt/min
    e. 30 gtt/min

49. Order "Aminophylline 50 mg/hr. The solution is 200 mg of aminophylline in 250 ml $\frac{1}{2}$ NSS." How many ml per hour are to be infused?

    _____   **49.** d

    a. 10 ml/hr
    b. 25.5 ml/hr
    c. 31 ml/hr
    d. 62.5 ml/hr
    e. 100 ml/hr

50. Order: "IV 1,000 cc PSS with 40,000 units of heparin to infuse at 75 ml/hr." What is the

    dose of heparin delivered every hour? _____   **50.** c

    a. 1,000 units
    b. 2,000 units
    c. 3,000 units
    d. 4,000 units
    e. 5,000 units

51. Biaxin is ordered for a 24 pound child. The recommended dose is 7.5 mg/kg every 12 hours. It comes 125 mg/5 ml. You would

    give _____ ml each dose.   **51.** b

    a. 2.1
    b. 3.3
    c. 4.1
    d. 4.5
    e. 5.0

52. Motrin is recommended for children at the dose 10 mg/kg/dose. It comes 40mg/ml. How much would you give to a 12 pound child?

_____

52. c

a. 0.6
b. 1.0
c. 1.4
d. 1.8
e. 2.1

---

53. Amoxicillin is ordered for a 13 pound infant. The recommended dose is 20 mg/kg/day in 3 divided doses. It comes as 125 mg/5 ml. You would give _____ ml each dose.

53. b

a. 1.0
b. 1.6
c. 2.0
d. 2.6
e. 5

---

54. Benadryl (diphenhydramine) is ordered for a 4 year old. The recommended dose is 6.25 mg every 4–6 hours for children 2 to 6 years old. It comes 12.5 mg/5 ml. How much would you give each dose? _____

54. a

a. 0.5 ml
b. 0.75 ml
c. 1 ml
d. 1.25 ml
e. 1.5 ml